T0294602

Pediatric Craniomaxillofacial Trauma

Editor

SRINIVAS M. SUSARLA

ORAL AND MAXILLOFACIAL SURGERY CLINICS OF NORTH AMERICA

www.oralmaxsurgery.theclinics.com

Consulting Editor
RUI P. FERNANDES

November 2023 • Volume 35 • Number 4

ELSEVIER

1600 John F. Kennedy Boulevard • Suite 1800 • Philadelphia, Pennsylvania, 19103-2899

http://www.oralmaxsurgery.theclinics.com

ORAL AND MAXILLOFACIAL SURGERY CLINICS OF NORTH AMERICA Volume 35, Number 4
November 2023 ISSN 1042-3699, ISBN-13: 978-0-443-18280-8

Editor: John Vassallo; j.vassallo@elsevier.com
Developmental Editor: Anita Chamoli

© 2023 Elsevier Inc. All rights reserved.

Oral and Maxillofacial Surgery Clinics of North America (ISSN 1042-3699) is published quarterly by Elsevier Inc., 360 Park Avenue South, New York, NY 10010-1710. Months of issue are February, May, August, and November. Business and Editorial Offices: 1600 John F. Kennedy Blvd., Suite 1800, Philadelphia, PA 19103-2899. Periodicals postage paid at New York, NY and additional mailing offices. Subscription prices are $409.00 per year for US individuals, $785.00 per year for US institutions, $100.00 per year for US students/residents, $483.00 per year for Canadian individuals, $941.00 per year for Canadian institutions, $100.00 per year for Canadian students/residents, $535.00 per year for international individuals, $941.00 per year for international institutions and $235.00 per year for international students/residents. To receive student/resident rate, orders must be accompanied by name or affiliated institution, date of term, and the *signature* of program/residency coordinator on institution letterhead. Orders will be billed at individual rate until proof of status is received. Foreign air speed delivery is included in all *Clinics* subscription prices. All prices are subject to change without notice. **POSTMASTER:** Send address changes to *Oral and Maxillofacial Surgery Clinics of North America,* Elsevier Periodicals **Customer Service, 11830 Westline Industrial Drive, St. Louis, MO 63146. Tel: 1-800-654-2452 (U.S. and Canada); 314-447-8871 (outside U.S. and Canada). Fax: 314-447-8029. E-mail: journalscustomerservice-usa@elsevier.com (for print support); journalsonlinesupport-usa@elsevier.com (for online support).**

Reprints. For copies of 100 or more, of articles in this publication, please contact the Commercial Reprints Department, Elsevier Inc., 360 Park Avenue South, New York, NY 10010-1710. Tel.: 212-633-3874; Fax: 212-633-3820; Email: reprints@elsevier.com.

Oral and Maxillofacial Surgery Clinics of North America is covered in *MEDLINE/PubMed (Index Medicus), Science Citation Index Expanded (SciSearch®), Journal Citation Reports/Science Edition,* and *Current Contents®/Clinical Medicine.*

Contributors

CONSULTING EDITOR

RUI P. FERNANDES, MD, DMD, FACS, FRCS(Ed)
Clinical Professor and Chief, Division of Head and Neck Surgery, Program Director, Head and Neck Oncologic Surgery and Microvascular Reconstruction Fellowship, Departments of Oral and Maxillofacial Surgery, Neurosurgery, and Orthopaedic Surgery and Rehabilitation, University of Florida Health Science Center, University of Florida College of Medicine, Jacksonville, Florida

EDITOR

SRINIVAS M. SUSARLA, DMD, MD, MPH, FACS, FAAP
Associate Professor of Oral and Maxillofacial Surgery and Plastic Surgery, University of Washington; Division Chief, Pediatric Oral and Maxillofacial Surgery, Craniofacial Center, Seattle Children's Hospital, Seattle, Washington

AUTHORS

SHELLY ABRAMOWICZ, DMD, MPH
Professor of Surgery, Division of Oral and Maxillofacial Surgery, Department of Surgery, Emory University School of Medicine, Children's Healthcare of Atlanta, Atlanta, Georgia

SUZANNE BARNES, DMD
Assistant Professor, Department of Oral and Maxillofacial Surgery, University of Louisville School of Dentistry, Louisville, Kentucky

APARNA BHAT, DMD, MD
Resident, Department of Oral and Maxillofacial Surgery, University of Washington School of Dentistry, University of Washington, Seattle, Washington

CRAIG B. BIRGFELD, MD
Associate Professor, Department of Surgery, Division of Plastic Surgery, University of Washington, Craniofacial Center, Seattle Children's Hospital, Seattle, Washington

RANDALL A. BLY, MD
Associate Professor, Department of Otolaryngology–Head and Neck Surgery, Seattle Childrens Hospital, Craniofacial Center, Department of Otolaryngology–Head and Neck Surgery, University of Washington, Seattle Children's Hospital, Seattle, Washington

RAQUEL CAPOTE, DMD, MSD, MPH
Assistant Professor of Oral and Maxillofacial Surgery, Vanderbilt University Medical Center,

Cleft and Craniofacial Program, Monroe Carell Jr. Children's Hospital at Vanderbilt, Nashville, Tennessee

SRINIVASA RAMA CHANDRA, BDS, MD, FDS, FIBCSOMS
Associate Professor and Program Director, OMFS-Head and Neck Oncology and Reconstructive Surgery, Oregon Health and Science University, Portland, Oregon

HANNAH C. COCKRELL, MD
Pediatric Surgery Equity Research Fellow, Department of Surgery, University of Washington, Division of Pediatric General and Thoracic Surgery, Seattle Children's Hospital, Seattle, Washington

MARK A. EGBERT, DDS, FACS
Associate Professor of Oral and Maxillofacial Surgery and Plastic Surgery, University of Washington, Oral and Maxillofacial Surgeon, Craniofacial Center, Seattle Children's Hospital, Seattle, Washington

RICHARD G. ELLENBOGEN, MD
Theodore S. Roberts Chair and Professor of Neurological Surgery, University of Washington School of Medicine, Seattle, Washington

MARK ENGELSTAD, DDS, MD
Associate Professor, Department of Oral Maxillofacial Surgery, Oregon Health and Science University, Portland, Oregon

RUSSELL E. ETTINGER, MD
Assistant Professor, Division of Plastic Surgery, Department of Surgery University of Washington, Craniofacial Center, Seattle Children's Hospital, Seattle, Washington

MICHAEL P. GRANT, MD, PhD, FACS
Division of Plastic and Reconstructive Surgery, R Adams Cowley Shock Trauma Center, University of Maryland Medical Center, Baltimore, Maryland

SARAH L.M. GREENBERG, MD, MPH
Assistant Professor of Surgery, Division of Pediatric General and Thoracic Surgery, Seattle Children's Hospital, Department of Surgery, University of Washington, Seattle, Washington

JEFFREY HAJIBANDEH, DDS, MD
Instructor, Harvard School of Dental Medicine, Staff Surgeon, Division of Oral and Maxillofacial Surgery, Director of Quality & Safety, Department of Oral & Maxillofacial Surgery, Massachusetts General Hospital, Boston, Massachusetts

BASHAR HASSAN, MD
Division of Plastic and Reconstructive Surgery, R Adams Cowley Shock Trauma Center, University of Maryland Medical Center, Department of Plastic and Reconstructive Surgery, Johns Hopkins Hospital, Baltimore, Maryland

ELIZABETH HOPKINS, MD
Instructor of Plastic and Reconstructive Surgery, Johns Hopkins University, Baltimore, Maryland

RICHARD A. HOPPER, MD, MS
Marlys C. Larson Chair and Professor of Surgery (Plastic), University of Washington School of Medicine, Surgical Director and Division Chief, Plastic and Craniofacial Surgery, Craniofacial Center, Seattle Children's Hospital, Seattle, Washington

MARCUS HWANG, DDS, MD
Resident, Department of Oral Maxillofacial Surgery, Oregon Health and Science University, Portland, Oregon

HITESH KAPADIA, DDS, PhD
Assistant Professor, Departments of Plastic Surgery and Orthodontics, Schools of Medicine and Dentistry, University of Washington; Division Chief, Craniofacial Center, Seattle Children's Hospital, Seattle, Washington

GEORGE M. KUSHNER, DMD, MD
Chairman and Professor, Department of Oral and Maxillofacial Surgery, University of Louisville School of Dentistry, Louisville, Kentucky

AMY LEE, MD
Professor of Neurological Surgery, University of Washington School of Medicine, Chief, Division of Pediatric Neurosurgery, Seattle Children's Hospital, Seattle, Washington

KEVIN C. LEE, DDS, MD
Fellow, of Oral and Maxillofacial Surgery, University at Buffalo, Department of Head and Neck/Plastic and Reconstructive Surgery, Roswell Park Comprehensive Cancer Center, Buffalo, New York

FAN LIANG, MD
Assistant Professor, Department of Plastic and Reconstructive Surgery, R Adams Cowley Shock Trauma Center, University of Maryland Medical Center, Medical Director, Johns Hopkins Hospital, Baltimore, Maryland

RACHEL LIM, DDS, MD
Resident, Department of Oral and Maxillofacial Surgery, University of Washington School of Dentistry, University of Washington, Seattle, Washington

G. NINA LU, MD
Assistant Professor, of Otolaryngology–Head and Neck Surgery, University of Washington, Seattle Children's Hospital, Seattle, Washington

SCOTT MANNING, MD
Professor, Department of Otolaryngology–Head and Neck Surgery, University of Washington School of Medicine; Chief, Division of Plastic Surgery, Department of Otolaryngology–Head and Neck Surgery, Seattle Childrens Hospital, Craniofacial Center, Seattle, Washington

MICHAEL R. MARKIEWICZ, DDS, MPH, MD, FAAP, FRCD(c), FACS
Professor and Chair, Department of Oral and Maxillofacial Surgery, University at Buffalo, Buffalo, New York

JEFFREY S. MARSCHALL, DMD, MD, MS
Assistant Professor, Department of Oral and Maxillofacial Surgery, University of Iowa Hospital and Clinics, Iowa City, Iowa

BENJAMIN B. MASSENBURG, MD
Division of Plastic and Reconstructive Surgery, Department of Surgery, University of Washington; Plastic Surgeon, Division of Plastic Surgery, Department of Otolaryngology–Head and Neck Surgery,

Seattle Childrens Hospital, Craniofacial Center, Seattle, Washington

MALIA MCAVOY, MD, MS
Resident, Department of Neurosurgery, University of Washington School of Medicine, Seattle, Washington

ZACHARY S. PEACOCK, DMD, MD, FACS
Chair, Department of Oral and Maxillofacial Surgery, Harvard School of Dental Medicine, Chief, Oral and Maxillofacial Surgery, Massachusetts General Hospital, Boston, Massachusetts

KATHRYN PRESTON, DDS, MS
Adjunct Professor, Department of Orthodontics, Arizona School of Dentistry and Oral Health, A.T. Still University; Craniofacial Orthodontist, Center for Cleft and Craniofacial Care, Phoenix Children's Hospital, Phoenix, Mesa, Arizona

MATTHEW J. RECKER, MD
Resident Physician, Department of Neurosurgery, Jacobs School of Medicine and Biomedical Sciences, State University of New York at Buffalo, Buffalo, New York

RENÉE REYNOLDS, MD
Clinical Associate Professor, Department of Neurosurgery, Jacobs School of Medicine and Biomedical Sciences, State University of New York at Buffalo, Buffalo, New York

SAMEER SHAKIR, MD
Assistant Professor, Department of Plastic Surgery, Medical College of Wisconsin; Plastic Surgeon, Children's Wisconsin, Milwaukee, Wisconsin

BARBARA SHELLER, DDS, MSD
Affiliate Professor of Orthodontics and Pediatric Dentistry, University of Washington School of Dentistry; Division Chief of Pediatric Dentistry, Department of Dentistry, Seattle Children's Hospital, Seattle, Washington

HARLYN K. SUSARLA, DMD, MPH
Affiliate Assistant Professor of Pediatric Dentistry, University of Washington School of Dentistry; Pediatric Dentist, Department of Dentistry, Seattle Children's Hospital, Seattle, Washington

SRINIVAS M. SUSARLA, DMD, MD, MPH, FACS, FAAP
Associate Professor of Oral and Maxillofacial Surgery and Plastic Surgery, University of Washington; Division Chief, Pediatric Oral and Maxillofacial Surgery, Craniofacial Center, Seattle Children's Hospital, Seattle, Washington

JEFFREY QUINN TAYLOR II, DMD
Resident in Training, Oral and Maxillofacial Surgery, Department of Surgery, Emory University School of Medicine, Atlanta, Georgia

PHILIP D. TOLLEY, MD
Resident Physician, Division of Plastic and Reconstructive Surgery, Department of Surgery, University of Washington; Plastic Surgeon, Division of Plastic Surgery, Department of Otolaryngology–Head and Neck Surgery, Seattle Childres Hospital, Craniofacial Center, Seattle, Washington

ROBIN YANG, DDS, MD
Director of Pediatric Plastic Surgery, Assistant Professor, Department of Plastic and Reconstructive Surgery, Johns Hopkins University, Baltimore, Maryland

Contents

Preface: Pediatric Craniomaxillofacial Trauma   **xiii**

Srinivas M. Susarla

General Care Considerations for the Pediatric Trauma Patient   **493**

Hannah C. Cockrell and Sarah L.M. Greenberg

Trauma is a leading cause of morbidity and mortality for children in the United States. Access to trauma care, injury burden, and outcomes following injury, are inequitable. There are many anatomic and physiologic differences between children and adults that affect injury patterns and necessary trauma treatment. The principles of advanced trauma life support (ATLS) should be used by clinicians in high-resource settings for the immediate in-hospital treatment of the injured child.

Craniofacial Growth and Development: A Primer for the Facial Trauma Surgeon   **501**

Raquel Capote, Kathryn Preston, and Hitesh Kapadia

Understanding craniofacial growth and development is important in the management of facial trauma in the growing pediatric patient. This manuscript is a review of craniofacial growth and development and clinical implications of pediatric facial fractures.

Epidemiology and Etiology of Facial Injuries in Children   **515**

Jeffrey Quinn Taylor II, Elizabeth Hopkins, Robin Yang, and Shelly Abramowicz

Pediatric Trauma results in over 8 million emergency department visits and 11,000 deaths annually. Unintentional injuries continue to be the leader in morbidity and mortality in pediatric and adolescent populations in the United States. More than 10% of all visits to pediatric emergency rooms (ER) present with craniofacial injuries. The most common etiologies for facial injuries in children and adolescence are motor vehicle accidents, assault, accidental injuries, sports injuries, nonaccidental injuries (eg, child abuse) and penetrating injuries. In the United States, head trauma secondary to abuse is the leading cause of mortality among non-accidental trauma in this population.

Intermaxillary Fixation in the Primary and Mixed Dentition   **521**

Jeffrey S. Marschall, Suzanne Barnes, and George M. Kushner

Anatomic differences of the primary dentition may hinder traditional methods of intermaxillary fixation. Furthermore, the presence of both the primary and permanent dentition can complicate establishing, and maintaining, the preinjury occlusion. The treating surgeon must be aware of these differences for optimal treatment outcomes. This article discusses and illustrates methods that facial trauma surgeons can use to establish intermaxillary fixation in children aged 12 years and younger.

Rigid Fixation of the Pediatric Facial Skeleton   529

Kevin C. Lee, Renée Reynolds, Matthew J. Recker, and Michael R. Markiewicz

> Pediatric facial fractures are uncommon, and fortunately, the majority can be managed with conservative measures. Rigid fixation of the pediatric facial skeleton can potentially be associated with delayed hardware issues and growth inhibition. When appropriate, resorbable fixation is most commonly used for this purpose. Titanium plates and screws are advantageous when rigid fixation is a priority because properly placed hardware that respects natural suture lines is not thought to significantly inhibit growth. Furthermore, titanium fixation may be removed following healing.

Dental and Dentoalveolar Injuries in the Pediatric Patient   543

Harlyn K. Susarla and Barbara Sheller

> Dental and dentoalveolar injuries are common in the pediatric population. Management is predicated on the type of tooth injured (primary or permanent), extent of injury, the dental and behavioral age of the patient, and ability of the patient to tolerate treatment. Although many dental injuries occur in isolation, a systematic evaluation of the patient is mandatory to confirm the absence of basal bone fractures of the maxilla or mandible, traumatic brain injury, cervical spine injury, and/or facial soft tissue injury. Long-term follow-up is paramount to achieving a functional occlusion and optimal dental health following injury.

Pediatric Mandible Fractures   555

Jeffrey Hajibandeh and Zachary S. Peacock

> The management of pediatric facial fractures requires several considerations by the treating surgeon. Pediatric facial fractures occur less commonly than in adults. Among fracture patterns in children, studies have repeatedly demonstrated that mandible fractures are the most common facial fracture particularly the condyle. Most fractures in children are amenable to nonsurgical or closed treatment; however, certain indications exist for open treatment. The literature describing epidemiology, treatment trends, and long-term outcomes are limited in comparison with adult populations. The purpose of the article is to review the etiology, workup, and management of mandible fractures in children

Pediatric Le Fort, Zygomatic, and Naso-Orbito-Ethmoid Fractures   563

Aparna Bhat, Rachel Lim, Mark A. Egbert, and Srinivas M. Susarla

> Fractures of the pediatric midface are infrequent, particularly in children in the primary dentition, due to the prominence of the upper face relative to the midface and mandible. With downward and forward growth of the face, there is an increasing frequency of midface injuries seen in children in the mixed and adult dentitions. Midface fracture patterns seen in young children are quite variable; those in children at or near skeletal maturity mimic patterns seen in adults. Non-displaced injuries can typically be managed with observation. Displaced fractures require treatment with appropriate reduction and fixation and longitudinal follow-up to evaluate growth.

Pediatric Nasal and Septal Fractures   577

Philip D. Tolley, Benjamin B. Massenburg, Scott Manning, G. Nina Lu, and Randall A. Bly

> Pediatric nasal bone and septal fractures represent a large number of craniofacial injuries in children each year. Due to their differences in anatomy and potential for growth and development, the management of these injuries varies slightly from

that of the adult population. As with most pediatric fractures, there is a bias toward less-invasive management to limit disruption to future growth. Often this includes closed reduction and splinting in the acute setting followed by open septorhino-plasty at skeletal maturity as needed. The overall goal of treatment is to restore the nose to its preinjury shape, structure, and function.

Pediatric Orbital Fractures   585

Bashar Hassan, Fan Liang, and Michael P. Grant

The unique anatomy and physiology of the growing craniofacial skeleton predispose children to different fracture patterns as compared to adults. Diagnosis and treatment of pediatric orbital fractures can be challenging. A thorough history and physical examination are essential for the diagnosis of pediatric orbital fractures. Physicians should be aware of symptoms and signs suggestive of trapdoor fractures with soft tissue entrapment including symptomatic diplopia with positive forced ductions, restricted ocular motility (regardless of conjunctival abnormalities), nausea/vomiting, bradycardia, vertical orbital dystopia, enophthalmos, and hypoglobus. Equivocal radiologic evidence of soft tissue entrapment should not withhold surgery. A multidisciplinary approach is recommended for the accurate diagnosis and proper management of pediatric orbital fractures.

Pediatric Cranial Vault and Skull Base Fractures   597

Malia McAvoy, Richard A. Hopper, Amy Lee, Richard G. Ellenbogen, and Srinivas M. Susarla

Cranial vault and skull base fractures in children are distinctly different from those seen in adults. Pediatric skull fractures have the benefit of greater capacity to remodel; however, the developing pediatric brain and craniofacial skeleton present unique challenges to diagnosis, natural history, and management. This article discusses the role of surgical treatment of these fractures, its indications, and techniques.

Pediatric Panfacial Fractures   607

Sameer Shakir, Russell E. Ettinger, Srinivas M. Susarla, and Craig B. Birgfeld

Pediatric panfacial trauma is a rare occurrence with poorly understood implications for the growing child. Treatment algorithms largely mirror adult panfacial protocols with notable exceptions including augmented healing and remodeling capacities that favor nonoperative management, limited exposure to avoid disruption of osseous suture and synchondroses growth centers, and creative fracture fixation techniques in the setting of an immature craniomaxillofacial skeleton. The following article provides a review of our institutional philosophy in the management of these challenges injuries with important anatomic, epidemiologic, examination, sequencing, and postoperative considerations.

Management of Soft Tissue Injuries in Children–A Comprehensive Review   619

Marcus Hwang, Mark Engelstad, and Srinivasa Rama Chandra

Airway injury, Ocular injury and neurovascular tissue damage, burns is all a spectrum of pediatric soft tissue injury complex. Soft tissue injuries to the head and neck area in children are challenging to manage, because these injuries significantly affect the child's overall health and development. Management of such injuries requires a multidisciplinary approach involving surgical and nonsurgical interventions and close collaboration among health care professionals, parents, and caregivers. This article reviews the various causes of injuries, specific considerations for each region of the head and neck, and approaches to the surgical management of soft tissue injuries in pediatric patients, including surgical and adjuvant therapies. Specific anatomic regions reviewed include the scalp/forehead, periorbital region, nose, cheeks, lips, ears, and neck/airway.Laceration repair in the growing pediatric populations may require revisions in the future. Facial soft tissue injuries are prone to poor cosmesis as in many occasions as may be constrained by available surgical specialists, thus proper multispecialty team approach along with surgical alignment and symmetry should be considered comprehensively.

ORAL AND MAXILLOFACIAL SURGERY CLINICS OF NORTH AMERICA

FORTHCOMING ISSUES

February 2024
Molecular, Therapeutic, and Surgical Updates on Head and Neck Vascular Anomalies
Srinivasa R. Chandra and Sanjiv Nair, *Editors*

May 2024
Gender Affirming Surgery
Russell E. Ettinger, *Editor*

August 2024
Pediatric Craniomaxillofacial Pathology
Srinivas M. Susarla, *Editor*

RECENT ISSUES

August 2023
Imaging of Common Oral Cavity, Sinonasal, and Skull Base Pathology
Dinesh Rao, *Editor*

May 2023
Diagnosis and Management of Oral Mucosal Lesions
Donald Cohen and Indraneel Bhattacharyya, *Editors*

February 2023
Global Perspective in Contemporary Orthognathic Surgery
Yiu Yan Leung, *Editor*

SERIES OF RELATED INTEREST

Atlas of the Oral and Maxillofacial Surgery Clinics
www.oralmaxsurgeryatlas.theclinics.com

Dental Clinics
www.dental.theclinics.com

THE CLINICS ARE NOW AVAILABLE ONLINE!
Access your subscription at:
www.theclinics.com

Preface
Pediatric Craniomaxillofacial Trauma

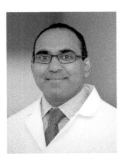

Srinivas M. Susarla, DMD, MD, MPH
Editor

This issue of the *Oral and Maxillofacial Surgery Clinics of North America* focuses on the contemporary management of craniomaxillofacial trauma in children and adolescents. Though somewhat less frequent than injuries seen in adults, facial injuries in children merit special considerations due to the anatomy and physiology of the pediatric facial skeleton as well as the impact that injuries and treatment may have on subsequent growth and development.

Effective care of the pediatric facial trauma patient requires close collaboration between emergency department and acute care providers, surgical specialists (craniomaxillofacial surgeons, pediatric surgeons, neurosurgeons) and primary care pediatric providers (pediatricians, pediatric dentists, orthodontists). We are very fortunate in this issue to have a diverse set of authors representing the array of specialties involved in the care of children who sustain facial injuries. There is no doubt that these clinical challenges are best managed multidisciplinary teams who work together not only to manage the physical and psychological issues patients (and their families) face in the acute setting but also to provide long-term follow-up care to monitor growth and development. The contributions in this issue have been meticulously crafted to demonstrate that message. I remain indebted to our expert authors, who have taken time away from their professional and personal commitments to provide outstanding contributions covering this expansive topic. It is my hope that this issue will serve as a high-yield reference for practitioners caring for this population across the spectrum of clincial contexts.

In addition to our contributors, there are a number of individuals who have helped this issue come to fruition and merit special recognition. Dr Rui Fernandes has been an outstanding friend and mentor and helped me define the scope of this subject and develop a product that is both comprehensive and accessible. John Vassallo's thoughtful guidance, rooted in an immense experience with the *Oral and Maxillofacial Surgery Clinics of North America*, allowed for a seamless process, from project inception to publication. Jessica Cañaberal worked to ensure that the process for contributors was straightforward and helped maintain the forward momentum needed to develop a high-quality issue on a strict timetable.

Finally, I would like to thank my wife, Dr Harlyn Susarla, for being a great life partner (and, in this context, a clinical partner as well). Her devotion to our family is matched by her devotion to the care of pediatric dental patients and is a model to emulate.

Srinivas M. Susarla, DMD, MD, MPH
Craniofacial Center
Seattle Children's Hospital
4800 Sand Point Way Northeast
Seattle, WA 98105, USA

E-mail address:
srinivas.susarla@seattlechildrens.org

oralmaxsurgery.theclinics.com

Oral Maxillofacial Surg Clin N Am 35 (2023) xiii
https://doi.org/10.1016/j.coms.2023.06.001
1042-3699/23/© 2023 Published by Elsevier Inc.

General Care Considerations for the Pediatric Trauma Patient

Hannah C. Cockrell, MD[a,b], Sarah L.M. Greenberg, MD, MPH[a,b],*

KEYWORDS

- Trauma • Injury • Pediatric • Health equity • ATLS • Pediatric surgery

KEY POINTS

- Trauma is a leading cause of morbidity and mortality for children and adolescents in the United States.
- Access to trauma care, and outcomes following injury, are inequitable.
- There are key anatomic and physiologic differences between children and adults that affect injury patterns, which can help guide appropriate care.

INTRODUCTION AND OVERVIEW

Injury is the leading cause of morbidity and mortality for children and adolescents in the United States.[1–7] Although reductions in deaths from some causes, such as motor vehicle collisions, have been realized over time, substantial and sustained increases have been seen in childhood mortality secondary to gun violence over the past decade.[4] Gross inequities are seen with the burden of injury, injury distribution, access to trauma care, and outcomes following injury for children in this country.[8,9] Injury affects the immediate and future health and welfare of children and their families, as well as the economic development and security of the communities in which they live.[1]

The purpose of this review is to provide an overview of pediatric trauma and general care considerations of the injured child for oral and maxillofacial care providers. This review discusses the epidemiology of injury in children and adolescents in the United States, outlines important anatomic and physiologic considerations in the injured child and how they may contribute to injury pattern and management, and delineates initial assessment and management strategies contained within the Advance Trauma Life Support (ATLS) model. It has an emphasis on initial hospital management within a well-resourced health system.

EPIDEMIOLOGY

Trauma is a leading cause of death and disability for children in the United States.[2–7] The Centers for Disease Control and Prevention (CDC) reported that unintentional injury–including motor vehicle collisions and falls–was the primary category of death for children spanning the ages of one and fourteen years old between 2018 and 2021, resulting in approximately 4.9 deaths per 100,000 population.[2] Assault by others was the 4th most common cause of death in this age group, followed by intentional self-harm.[2] Firearm-related injury, which can fall within all of these categories, is rapidly rising and is currently the singular leading cause of death among children and adolescents in the United States.[4] Children living in communities in urban settings, as well as those in communities

a Division of Pediatric General and Thoracic Surgery, Seattle Children's Hospital, 4800 Sand Point Way Northeast, Seattle, WA 98105, USA; b Department of Surgery, University of Washington, Box 356410, 1959 NE Pacific Street, Seattle, WA 98195, USA
* Corresponding author. Division of Pediatric General and Thoracic Surgery, Seattle Children's Hospital, 4800 Sand Point Way Northeast, Seattle, WA 98105.
E-mail address: Sarah.Greenberg@seattlechildrens.org

Oral Maxillofacial Surg Clin N Am 35 (2023) 493–499
https://doi.org/10.1016/j.coms.2023.05.003

with high levels of socioeconomic disadvantage, suffer a disproportionate burden of penetrating trauma.[10–12] For every child that dies secondary to injury, there are approximately 25 children hospitalized and 925 treated in emergency departments.[3]

Despite the high prevalence of morbidity and mortality from trauma for children, significant inequities exist in access to centers able to care for such injuries, injury burden, and outcomes resulting from physical trauma.[8,9] For example, children experience improved outcomes when treated for injury at pediatric trauma centers, but only 22.3% of injured children in the United States receive care at such facilities [Burdick]. Only half of the US pediatric population can reach a pediatric trauma center by ground transportation within the golden hour following injury, with disparate access seen when stratified by race, ethnicity, socioeconomic characteristics and rurality.[9,11] Understanding the systems, structures, actions, and behaviors that create and perpetuate these inequities is critical for trauma prevention and treatment of children with injuries.

PRINCIPLES OF INITIAL IN-HOSPITAL MANAGEMENT WITH ADVANCED TRAUMA LIFE SUPPORT (ATLS)

The principles ATLS can be used by clinicians for the immediate in-hospital treatment of the injured child, allowing for rapid identification and treatment of life-threatening injuries.[13] This includes prompt assessment of the patient's condition, resuscitation, stabilization, and determination of the need for and facilitation of transfer based on patient status and facility resources.[13] The principles of initial assessment and management from the 10th edition of ATLS, with the specific consideration of the care of children, are reviewed in the paragraphs to follow.

The primary survey

Initial assessment and resuscitation of the injured child with the identification of life-threatening conditions can be done via a prioritized sequence using a primary survey.[13] This survey incorporates the ABCDEs of trauma care: airway, breathing, circulation, disability, and exposure:[13]

- Airway: Establishing/maintaining airway patency, including cervical spine immobilization.
  Airway assessment can be done by evaluating the patient's ability to speak or cry. It includes looking for signs of airway obstruction, identifying obvious facial, trachea or laryngeal fractures, and

suctioning of blood or secretions from the oropharynx. This may require the establishment of a definitive airway. Cervical spine motion should be limited with the assumption that a cervical spine injury may exist.

- Breathing: Ensuring adequate oxygenation and ventilation.

Breathing can be assessed by looking at chest wall excursion, assessing jugular venous distension and tracheal position, listening to breath sounds, and through the ability of the patient to generate air movement to speak or cry. Life-threatening injuries impairing ventilation, such as a tension pneumothorax, open pneumothorax, or massive pneumothorax, will need to be identified and treated during this stage such as via thoracic decompression.

- Circulation: Establishing effective circulation, including hemorrhage control and vascular access.

Circulation can be assessed by feeling for pulses, evaluating skin perfusion through capillary refill and extremity warmth and color, and considering the level of consciousness as a measure of cerebral perfusion. Hemorrhage is the primary cause of preventable death following injury. Massive external hemorrhage can be controlled with direct pressure and at times cautious tourniquet use. Internal hemorrhage should be considered within the chest, abdomen, retroperitoneum, pelvis and long bones. Temporary management may include the placement of a pelvic stabilizing device or extremity splints. Vascular assess should be established, typically with two large bore IVs, blood samples sent, and volume resuscitation maintained.

- Disability: Assessing neurologic status, including spine immobilization.
  Disability can be reviewed by evaluating the level of consciousness and rapid neurologic evaluation. This can be done by looking at the pupillary size and reaction and using a tool such as the GCS (Glasgow Coma Scale) to determine the level of consciousness (Table 1).
- Exposure and Environment: Preparing for a full exam while maintaining warmth.

Exposure can be obtained through the removal of patient clothing while warmth can be preserved or supported through external warming devices such as blankets and heating lights to prevent hypothermia.

Table 1
Pediatric glasgow coma scale

	Infants	Children	Score
Eye Opening	Open spontaneously	Open spontaneously	4
	Open to verbal stimuli	Open to verbal stimuli	3
	Open to pain	Open to pain	2
	No response	No response	1
Verbal Response	Coos, babbles	Oriented, appropriate	5
	Irritable cries	Confused	4
	Cries in response to pain	Inappropriate words	3
	Moans in response to pain	Incomprehensible words or sounds	2
	No response	No response	1
Motor Response	Moves spontaneously and purposefully	Follows commands	6
	Withdraws to touch	Localizes to pain	5
	Withdraws to pain	Withdraws in response to pain	4
	Flexor posturing to pain	Flexor posturing to pain	3
	Extensor posturing to pain	Extensor posturing to pain	2
	No response	No response	1

Data from References[24,25]

Adjuncts to the primary survey can include continuous electrocardiography, pulse oximetry, measurement of end tidal CO2, and arterial blood gas (ABG) measurements. X-rays of the chest and pelvis, focused the assessment of sonography for trauma (FAST), and diagnostic peritoneal lavage (DPL) can be obtained. Additional labs can be completed, and gastric and urinary catheters can be placed.

The need for immediate transfer or immediate operative intervention should also be determined during the primary survey.

The secondary survey

After the completion of the primary survey with improvement or normalization of vital signs and ongoing resuscitation, care providers can then move on to the secondary survey. The secondary survey is a complete examination of the patient, including a head-to-toe physical exam and determination of a history if possible. Depending on the patient's age and injury status, the history may need to come from family members of the injured child. The pneumonic AMPLE can be used to elicit the patient's medical history and details of injury.

- *A*llergies
- *M*edications
- *P*ast illness
- *L*ast meal
- *E*vents of the injury
A complete, head-to-toe physical exam should be completed, including log-rolling the patient.

Adjuncts to the secondary survey can include additional radiographs, CT scans, contrast urography, angiography, ultrasonography, bronchoscopy, esophagoscopy, and additional labs. Continuous monitoring of vital signs (**Table 2**) and urinary output in important, as is adequate pain management.

Re-evaluation of the patient should occur frequently to note any changes or previously undiscovered injuries. Any decline in patient status should prompt a return to and repeat of the primary survey.

Patient disposition, whether that be transfer to another facility, transfer to the operating room for surgical intervention, admission to the floor or ICU, or discharge home, should be decided. A summary of these ATLS principles for children can be found in **Table 3**.

PEDIATRIC-SPECIFIC ANATOMY AND PHYSIOLOGY

Multiple anatomic and physiologic differences exist between children and adults that affect injury patterns and trauma treatment for children.[14–17] In general, compared to adults, children have or experience the following.

High frequency of multi-system injury and polytrauma

Children have a smaller body mass than adults. Trauma therefore imparts increased energy per unit surface area to their bodies. In addition, children have less protective fat, muscle, and soft

Table 2
Vital signs in children

Heart Rate (Beats/min)			Respiratory Rate (Breaths/min)	
Age	Awake	Asleep	Age	Normal
Neonate (<28d)	100–205	90–160	Infant (<1 y)	30–53
Infant (1–12 mo)	100–190			
Toddler (1–2 y)	98–140	80–120	Toddler (1–2 y)	22–37
Preschool (3–5 y)	80–120	65–100	Preschool (3–5 y)	20–28
School-age (6–11 y)	75–118	58–90	School-age (6–11 y)	18–25
Adolescent (12–15 y)	60–100	50–90	Adolescent (12–15 y)	12–20

Blood Pressure (mm Hg)				
Age		Systolic Pressure	Diastolic Pressure	Mean Arterial Pressure
Birth (12 h)	< 1 kg	39–59	16–36	28–42
	3 kg	60–76	31–45	48–57
Neonate (96 h)		67–84	35–53	45–60
Infant (1–12 mo)		72–104	37–56	50–62
Toddler (1–2 y)		86–106	42–63	49–62
Preschool (3–5 y)		89–112	46–72	58–69
School-age (6–9 y)		97–115	57–76	66–72
Preadolescent (10–11y)		102–120	61–80	71–79
Adolescent (12–15 y)		110–131	64–83	73–84

Data from References[26,27]

tissue than many adults and a less calcified (and therefore less protective) skeleton. These factors lead to a high incidence of multi-system trauma with a greater incidence of abdominal, chest, and spinal cord fracture without associated bony injury or external injury. The presence of bony fractures in a child indicates massive energy transfer, and providers should be aware of the high likelihood of serious associated injuries.

High risk of hypothermia

Body surface area to body mass ratio decreases as an individual ages. Children also have high metabolic rates and minimal subcutaneous tissue. These factors put them at high risk of heat loss, which can affect response to interventions and outcomes following injury. Close regulation of body temperature with various warming devices and strategies including blankets, Bair Huggers, heat lamps, warmed IVF and heated inhaled gases and treatments is important.

Rapid decompensation

Compared to adults, children have abundant physiology reserve and compensatory mechanisms. They manifest fewer signs of hypovolemia compared to adults, despite significant volume depletion. Changes in extremity perfusion or

pulses, and tachycardia, which could also be secondary to many other causes such as pain or fear, may be the only signs of shock.[18] A 30% decrease in circulating blood volume may occur before a decrease in systolic blood pressure is seen.[13] Therefore, when physiologic decompensation does happen, it tends to be fast and severe.

Additional key anatomic and physiologic considerations

In addition, the oropharyngeal soft tissues in a child are larger than in an adult. The larynx tends to be more anterior and cephalad and the epiglottis may be floppy. These differences can make visualization more difficult during intubation. Children have a short tracheal length, increasing the risk of right-mainstem intubation, as well as endotracheal tube (ETT) dislodgement. Finally, the cricoid ring is the narrowest part of a child's airway, which could result in an ETT passing the vocal cords but getting stuck at the cricoid.

Children have large heads in relation to the size of their bodies. When supine, this can lead to cervical spine flexion and buckling of the posterior pharynx. To compensate for these differences, airway maintenance, and cervical spine neutrality

Table 3
Summary of ATLS protocol for pediatric trauma

Primary Survey	
Airway	Establish and maintain airway patency, including cervical spine immobilization • Look for signs of airway obstruction • Identify obvious facial, tracheal, or laryngeal fractures • Establish a definitive airway if indicated
Breathing	Ensure adequate oxygenation and ventilation • Assess chest wall excursion, jugular venous distension, and tracheal position • Auscultate breath sounds • Identify and treat life-threatening injuries impairing ventilation including tension pneumothorax or open pneumothorax
Circulation	Establish effective circulation, including hemorrhage control and vascular access • Assess pulses and evaluate extremity color and warmth • Control external hemorrhage with direct pressure or judicious use of tourniquets • Internal hemorrhage should be considered within the chest, abdomen, retroperitoneum, pelvis, and long bones. • Vascular access should be established with two large bore IVs. • Balanced blood product resuscitation should be initiated in the setting of hemorrhage.
Disability	Assess neurological status, including spine immobilization • Evaluate the level of consciousness and perform a rapid neurologic evaluation using the Pediatric Glasgow Coma Scale.
Exposure and environment	Prepare for a full exam while maintaining warmth • Remove patient clothing to perform a head-to-toe exam and evaluate for missed injuries. • Use blankets, heating lights, and radiant warmers to prevent hypothermia.
Secondary Survey	
Allergies	Determine relevant medication and food allergies, especially allergies to betadine and shellfish prior to the administration of iodinated contrast for computed tomography scans
Medications	Perform a medication reconciliation to ensure that critical medications are resumed upon hospital admission and to avoid medication cross-reactivity
Past illness	Elicit past medical history, including the history of bleeding diathesis
Last meal	Determine the time of last oral intake to assess aspiration risk and need for rapid sequence intubation if the patient requires airway protection, mechanical ventilation, or general anesthesia for operative intervention
Events of the injury	Obtain details of the event including the mechanism of injury and loss of consciousness

can be supported by placing padding, such as a blanket, under the child's torso. Children's large head-body ratio, combined with thinner cranial bones and a relatively smaller subarachnoid space puts children at high risk of head injury.[13,15]

Compared to adults, children have lower functional residual capacity, higher oxygen metabolism, and more rapid respiratory fatigue. These things put them at higher risk of hypoxia and respiratory decline.

ADDITIONAL CONSIDERATIONS FOR THE INJURED CHILD

Approximation of the weight of a child is critical to help guide resuscitation, determine appropriate vital signs (see **Table 2**), identify proper equipment sizes and direct apt drug dosing. The Broselow Pediatric Emergency Tape is a color-coded, length-based measure that utilizes a child's height to determine their weight. The Broselow tape includes suggested drug doses, fluid volumes and sizes for supplies and equipment.

It is critical that the care provider know age-appropriate vital signs in order to guide appropriate oxygenation, ventilation, and circulatory support (see **Table 2**).

CONSIDERATION FOR CHILD ABUSE OR MALTREATMENT

When caring for injured children, care providers should be aware of the risk of non-accidental trauma (NAT), or child abuse or maltreatment.[19] The CDC defines child abuse and neglect as any preventable act of commission or omission by a caregiver that results in harm, potential harm or threat of harm to a child.[20] Child abuse and neglect are quite common in the United States.[20] Approximately 1 in 7 children have experienced abuse or neglect over the past year. In 2020, at least 1750 children died of abuse and neglect in the US.[20] Despite this, care providers frequently fail to identify child abuse.[21–23] Concern for child abuse or maltreatment should increase with discrepant or inconsistent findings on history or physical examination, delayed presentation, prior injuries, or injuries that do not align with a child's developmental stage.[19]

SUMMARY/DISCUSSION

Injury affects the lives, health, and wellbeing of many children in the United States. Significant inequities exist with injury burden, access to trauma care, and outcomes following injury. Understanding key physiologic and anatomic differences between children and adults can help guide the management of injury. ATLS, when used with certain differences applicable to children, can be used for the initial assessment and management of trauma

CLINICS CARE POINTS

- In high-resource settings, the principles of Advanced Trauma Life Support (ATLS), with the consideration of the characteristics of children, should be used for the immediate in-hospital treatment injured children.

- There are many anatomic and physiologic differences between children and adults that affect injury pattern, presentation, and necessary treatment of injured children.
- Understanding of the systems, structures, behaviors and actions that generate and perpetuate inequities in injury burden, access to trauma care, and outcomes following injury are necessary for the prevention and treatment of injury in children.
- Child abuse or maltreatment should be considered when evaluating an injured child.

REFERENCES

1. American Academy of Pediatrics Section on Orthopaedics, American Academy of Pediatrics Committee on Pediatric Emergency Medicine, American Academy of Pediatrics Section on Critical Care, et al. Management of Pediatric Trauma. Pediatrics 2008;121(4):849–54.
2. CDC Wonder. Available at: https://wonder.cdc.gov. Accessed April 29, 2023.
3. Child Injury. Vital Signs. Centers for Disease Control and Prevention. Available at: https://www.cdc.gov/vitalsigns/childinjury/index.html. Accessed April 29, 2023.
4. Goldstick JE, Cunningham RM, Carter PM. Current causes of death in children and adolescents in the United States. N Engl J Med 2022;386(20):1955–6.
5. GBD Compare. Institute for Health Metrics and Evaluation. 2019. Available at: https://vizhub.healthdata.org/gbd-compare/. Accessed April 29, 2023.
6. Leading Causes of Death and Injury. Injury Prevention & Control. Centers for Disease Control and Prevention. Published 2023. Available at: https://www.cdc.gov/injury/wisqars/LeadingCauses.html. Accessed April 29, 2023.
7. Cunningham RM, Walton MA, Carter PM. The major causes of death in children and adolescents in the United States. N Engl J Med 2018;379(25):2468–75.
8. Newgard CD, Lin A, Olson LM, et al. Evaluation of emergency department pediatric readiness and outcomes among US trauma centers. JAMA Pediatr 2021;175(9):947–56.
9. Burdick KJ, Lee LK, Mannix R, et al. Racial and ethnic disparities in access to pediatric trauma centers in the United states: a geographic information systems analysis. Ann Emerg Med 2023;81(3):325–33.
10. Trinidad S, Brokamp C, Sahay R, et al. Children from disadvantaged neighborhoods experience disproportionate injury from interpersonal violence. J Pediatr Surg 2023;58(3):545–51.

11. Polcari AM, Hoefer LE, Callier K, et al. Social vulnerability index is strongly associated with urban pediatric firearm violence: an analysis of five major U.S. cities. J Trauma Acute Care 2023. https://doi.org/10.1097/ta.0000000000003896. Publish Ahead of Print.

12. Stevens J, Reppucci ML, Pickett K, et al. Using the social vulnerability index to examine disparities in surgical pediatric trauma patients. J Surg Res 2023;287:55–62.

13. American College of Surgeons Committee on Trauma. ATLS Advanced Trauma Life Support. 10th edition. Chicago, IL: American College of Surgeons; 2018.

14. Mikrogianakis A, Grant V. The Kids Are Alright: Pediatric Trauma Pearls. Emerg Med Clin North Am 2018;36(1):237–57.

15. Kissoon N, Dreyer J, Walia M. Pediatric trauma: differences in pathophysiology, injury patterns and treatment compared with adult trauma. Cmaj Can Medical Assoc J J De L'association Medicale Can. 1990;142(1):27–34.

16. Kenefake ME, Swarm M, Walthall J. Nuances in pediatric trauma. Emerg Med Clin 2013;31(3):627–52.

17. Overly FL, Wills H, Valente JH. 'Not just little adults' - a pediatric trauma primer. R I Med J (2013) 2014; 97(1):27–30.

18. Acker SN, Kulungowski AM. Error traps and culture of safety in pediatric trauma. Semin Pediatr Surg 2019;28(3):183–8.

19. Escobar MA, Wallenstein KG, Christison-Lagay ER, et al. Child abuse and the pediatric surgeon: A position statement from the Trauma Committee, the Board of Governors and the Membership of the American Pediatric Surgical Association. J Pediatr Surg 2019;54(7):1277–85.

20. Child Abuse and Neglect Prevention. Violence Prevention. Centers for Disease Control and Prevention. Published April 6, 2022. Available at: https://www.cdc.gov/violenceprevention/childabuseandneglect/index.html?CDC_AA_refVal=https%3A%2F%2Fwww.cdc.gov%2Fviolenceprevention%2Fchildmaltreatment%2Findex.html. Accessed April 29, 2023.

21. Jenny C, Hymel KP, Ritzen A, et al. Analysis of missed cases of abusive head trauma. JAMA 1999;281(7):621–6.

22. Ravichandiran N, Schuh S, Bejuk M, et al. Delayed identification of pediatric abuse-related fractures. Pediatrics 2010;125(1):60–6.

23. Sheets LK, Leach ME, Koszewski IJ, et al. Sentinel Injuries in Infants Evaluated for Child Physical Abuse. Pediatrics 2013;131(4):701–7.

24. Emergency Department Clinical Pathway for the Evaluation/Treatment of Children with Acute Head Trauma. Available at: https://www.chop.edu/clinical-pathway/head-trauma-acute-clinical-pathway. Accessed May 16, 2023.

25. Modified Glasgow Coma Scale for Infants and Children. Available at: https://www.merckmanuals.com/professional/SearchResults?query=modified+Glasgow+coma+scale+for+infants+and+children. Accessed May 16, 2023.

26. Novak C, Gill P. Pediatric Vital Signs Reference Chart. Available at: https://www.pedscases.com/sites/default/files/Vitals%20Chart_PedsCases%20Notes.pdf. Accessed May 16, 2023.

27. Topjian AA, Raymond TT, Atkins D, et al. Part 4: Pediatric basic and advanced life support: 2020 American heart association guidelines for cardiopulmonary resuscitation and emergency cardiovascular care. Circulation 2020;142(16_suppl_2):S469–523.

Craniofacial Growth and Development
A Primer for the Facial Trauma Surgeon

Raquel Capote, DMD, MSD, MPH[a,b,*], Kathryn Preston, DDS, MS[c,d],
Hitesh Kapadia, DDS, PhD[e,f,g]

KEYWORDS

- Craniofacial • Maxillofacial • Craniomaxillofacial • Facial • Pediatric • Growth and development
- Trauma • Fractures

KEY POINTS

- The craniofacial complex follows a cephalocaudal gradient of development. The skeleton grows differentially with different regions reaching adult dimensions at different times.
- Trauma to growth centers and growth sites during childhood can disrupt normal development. Intraoperative soft tissue damage, periosteal stripping, scar formation, and rigid fixation may also affect facial growth.
- The cranial vault after age 5 years and the orbit after age 7 years are generally of adult size and definitive reconstruction may be achieved. The maxilla, mandible, and nose do not achieve their adult dimensions until the adolescent pubertal growth spurt.
- Surgical treatment before skeletal maturity is less predictable and may require reoperation following skeletal maturation.
- It is critical to educate the patient/family on the potential for growth disturbances with long-term follow-up recommended until growth is completed.

INTRODUCTION

The craniofacial complex comprises the neurocranium, face, and oral apparatus, representing a morphologic and multifunctional region fundamental to being human. Structures develop through a dynamic process that begins in utero and reply upon complex temporally and spatially coordinated tissue interactions.[1] Craniofacial growth is characterized by cephalocaudal and allometric patterns.[2] Growth of tissues such as bone, cartilage, and muscle as well as highly specialized organs such as the brain and teeth contribute to the development of structures and creation of spaces supporting multiple functions.

The process of craniofacial growth is controlled by genetics, influenced by environmental factors.[3] Trauma can lead to dysmorphology as a result of the disruptive injury, secondary to the treatment, and/or subsequent growth and development.[4] The pediatric craniofacial complex exhibits distinct anatomic and physiologic differences compared to adults. It is important to identify not only the most appropriate intervention but the

[a] Department of Oral and Maxillofacial Surgery, Vanderbilt University Medical Center, Nashville, TN, USA; [b] Cleft and Craniofacial Program, Monroe Carell Jr. Children's Hospital at Vanderbilt, Nashville, TN, USA; [c] Center for Cleft and Craniofacial Care, Phoenix Children's Hospital, Phoenix, AZ, USA; [d] Department of Orthodontics, Arizona School of Dentistry & Oral Health, A.T. Still University, Mesa, AZ, USA; [e] Craniofacial Center, Seattle Children's Hospital, Seattle, WA, USA; [f] Division of Plastic Surgery, Department of Surgery, University of Washington, Seattle, WA, USA; [g] Department of Orthodontics, School of Dentistry, University of Washington, Seattle, WA, USA

* Corresponding author. Department of Oral and Maxillofacial Surgery, Vanderbilt University Medical Center, T-4323A Medical Center North, 1161 21st Avenue South Nashville, TN 37232-2596.
E-mail address: raquel.capote@vumc.org

Oral Maxillofacial Surg Clin N Am 35 (2023) 501–513
https://doi.org/10.1016/j.coms.2023.04.007

optimal time to surgically intervene for best outcome while minimizing detrimental impacts on subsequent growth. An understanding of craniofacial growth and development is critical to the management of pediatric facial trauma.

CORE CONCEPTS OF NORMAL GROWTH AND DEVELOPMENT
Concept 1: Growth Pattern

Craniofacial growth is expressed as a patterned series of changes in size, shape, and location.[5] At birth, the head is large in relation to the rest of the body and the cranium is disproportionately large relative to the face, following a cephalocaudal growth gradient and reflecting the dominance of brain development.[1] The newborn skull is given over to the neurocranium. The eyes, outgrowths of the forebrain, are relatively large. The midface and lower third of the face are diminutive and take a more retruded position (**Fig. 1**). With growth and development, the face "catches up" to cranial development, increasing susceptibility to midface and mandibular trauma.

Concept 2: Differential Development and Maturation

The complexity and diversity of the skull arises because the constituent bones enlarge differentially.[1] Facial growth occurs in 3 planes with the transverse dimension completed first, followed by completion of horizontal growth, and finally by vertical facial growth that continues into adulthood.[6–9] The facial region demonstrates variation in growth rates during development (**Table 1**[10–18] and **Fig. 2**). In particular, the mandible exhibits rapid growth around puberty. Surgical treatment performed before skeletal maturity is less predictable and may require reoperation following skeletal maturation.[14]

Concept 3: Mechanisms of Bone Growth: Drift and Displacement

There are 2 main mechanisms by which bone growth occurs: (1) drift (surface remodeling) through bone formation on one side and resorption on the other that produce a change in the size and shape of the bone and result in a change in location in the direction of external bony deposition; (2) displacement (translation) is the movement of the whole bone as a unit to a new location caused by the growth of adjacent structures. The overall direction of growth is the cumulative effect of displacement and drift[19] (**Fig. 3**).

Concept 4: Growth Centers versus Growth Sites

Fundamental to the understanding of craniofacial growth is an appreciation of growth centers and growth sites.[20,21] Areas of the growing skeleton that are primarily under the control of heredity are referred to as growth centers. Growth centers exhibit intrinsic, independent growth potential and active tissue separating force. Examples are synchondroses uniting endochondral bones in the cranial base and the nasal septal cartilage.

In contrast, a growth site is an area of skeletal growth that occurs secondarily and grows in compensatory fashion due to growth in a proximate location. Growth sites exhibit passive filling-in and/or remodeling in response to extrinsic forces or functional demands imposed by adjacent structures. This concept falls closely in line with the functional matrix theory. The brain, eye, and tooth may be considered the functional matrix of the cranial vault, orbits, and alveolus, respectively. The sutures connecting intramembranous bones found in the cranial vault and face and the periosteum are growth sites. It has been previously believed that the mandibular condyle is a primary

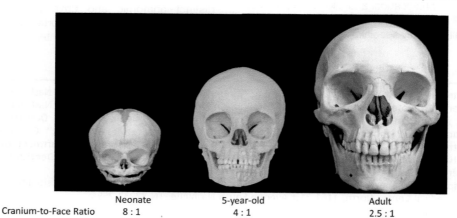

	Neonate	5-year-old	Adult
Cranium-to-Face Ratio	8 : 1	4 : 1	2.5 : 1

Fig. 1. Comparison between neonate and adult skull.

Table 1
Average percentage growth completion of various craniofacial structures

	Average % of Growth Completed by Age 1	Average % of Growth Completed by Age 5	Average Age at Maturity in Years
Cranial vault	84–88	93–96	Males: 14–15 Female: 13–14
Orbits	77–86	87–93	Males/females: 7 variable
Zygoma	72–74	83–86	Males: 15 Female: 13
Maxilla	75–80	85	Males: 16 Female: 14
Mandible	60–70	74–85	Males: 18–20 Female: 14–16

Data from Refs[10–18].

growth center although now the condyle is not credited as the sole determinate of mandibular growth potential. It is considered a growth site that is necessary for mandibular development and is influenced by intrinsic and extrinsic factors.[22]

NEUROCRANIUM

The neurocranium is the part of the skull that encloses the brain and includes the cranial base and cranial vault.

Cranial Base

The cranial base forms the inferior aspect of the cranium and provides a platform from which the face grows.[1] At birth, the cranial base is short and the spheno-ethmoidal synchondrosis (SES) and the spheno-occipital synchondrosis (SOS) are patent (**Fig. 4**). Bidirectional growth occurs interstitially at the cartilaginous joints located between 2 bones of endochondral origin[23] (**Fig. 5**). The SES and SOS are growth centers and are major contributors to anteroposterior growth of the cranial base and

displacement of the face. The maxilla articulates with the anterior cranial base and the mandible articulates with the temporal bone. Growth at the SES displaces the facial skeleton forward relative to the braincase. As the SES grows and elongates the anterior cranial base, the cranial vault expands and the ethmoid, zygomatic and palatine bones elongate, thereby increasing the size of the orbits and midface. As the SOS grows and elongates the middle cranial fossa, it displaces the glenoid fossa in the temporal bone posteriorly and inferiorly[24,25] while moving the face forward away from the vertebral column. This deepens the nasopharynx, creating more space for airway, muscles of mastication and room for growth of the ascending ramus of the mandible.

The greatest rate of increase in cranial base length and decrease in cranial base angulation occurs during the first 2 to 3 postnatal years.[26] The anterior cranial base is closer to its adult size than the posterior cranial base throughout postnatal growth. The SES fuses at about 7 years of age whereas the SOS continues to grow through adolescence. The SOS is the last synchondroses

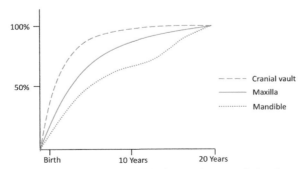

Fig. 2. Growth of the cranial vault, maxilla, and mandible from infancy to skeletal maturity. The cranial vault reaches maturity well before the midface and is followed by the mandible.

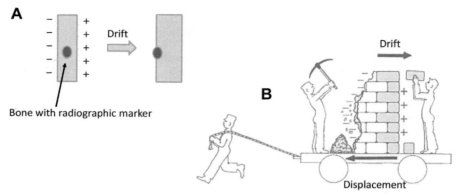

Fig. 3. Mechanisms of bone growth: drift and displacement. (*A*) Drift (surface remodeling). (*B*) Drift and displacement can occur in the same direction or in opposite directions as illustrated. (*From* Enlow D, Hans M. *Essentials of facial growth*. W. B. Saunders; 1996. (Figure 3B).)

of the cranial base to fuse with closure time occurring in girls at approximately 13 to 15 years of age and in boys around 15 to 17 years of age.[27] Once growth in the synchondroses ceases, the cartilage is replaced by bone to form synostoses.

Cranial Vault

The calvaria or cranial vault, together with the cranial base, encase and protect the brain. Like the cranial base, the most rapid postnatal expansion of the calvaria is during the first 2 years after birth.[23] However, unlike the cranial base, cranial sutures connecting the intramembranous bones of the calvaria are growth sites.[20]

The cranial vault is composed of paired frontal and parietal bones, the squamous parts of the temporal bone, and interparietal part of occipital bone that are separated by unossified sutures of fibrous connective tissues (**Fig. 6**). The cranial vault enlarges primarily as a result of compensatory growth at the sutural bone fronts stimulated by expansile growth of the neural elements.

Growth proceeds rapidly during the first 24 months after birth, secondary to the brain doubling in volume in the first 6 months and again by the second birthday.[28] The sutures normally remain patent and actively growing to keep pace as the brain expands. By age 5 years, the cranium is 90% of adult size.[15] After age 7 years, bony apposition on the outer surface of the frontal bone and development of the frontal sinus drifts the frontal bone and root of nose anteriorly.[23] The frontal sinuses that are absent at birth begin to develop at age 2 years, are radiographically detectable around age 6 to 7 years, and reach their full size after puberty.[29]

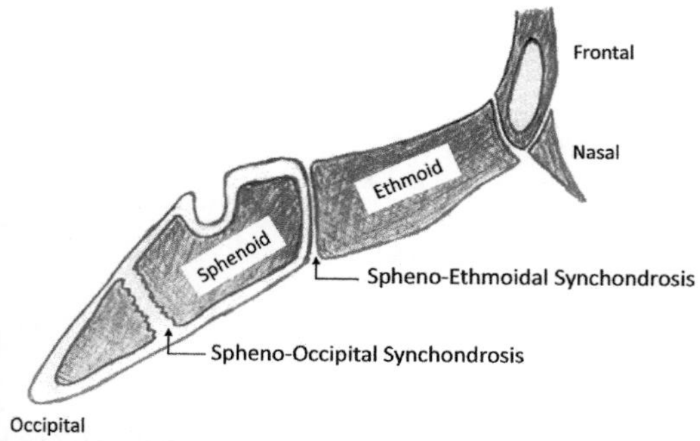

At birth, bones of the vault are thin, malleable, and unilaminar. As displacement of the individual flat bones of the cranial vault takes place, compensatory bone growth occurs at the sutures and by surface remodeling of the outer and inner cortex of the skull. An intervening diploë layer of spongy cancellous bone appears around age 4 years. By adulthood, the calvarial bones are thicker, rigid, and trilaminar. The calvaria bones remain separated by thin, periosteum-lined sutures for many years, eventually fusing in adult life.[30]

FACE

The face incorporates different anatomic and functional spaces and is composed of numerous individual bones, several of which are paired and most developing intramembranously. The anatomy of the face is divided into 3 main regions: upper, middle (midface), and lower (mandible).

Upper Face

The upper face contains the forehead, eyes, and temporal region. The orbit is composed of bones from the cranium (frontal, sphenoid, ethmoid, lacrimal) and nasomaxillary complex (maxillary, zygomatic, and palatine bones). The sutures

Frontal

Nasal

Ethmoid

Sphenoid

Spheno-Ethmoidal Synchondrosis

Spheno-Occipital Synchondrosis

Occipital

Fig. 4. Synchondroses.

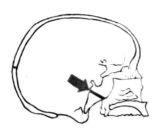

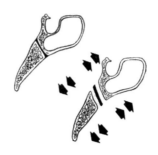

Fig. 5. Schematic drawing of a mid-sagittal view of the cranial base showing the spheno-occipital synchondrosis. Diagrammatic representation of the spheno-occipital synchondrosis. The spheno-ethmoidal synchondrosis, not shown, and the spheno-occipital synchondrosis exhibit a "bidirectional" pattern of growth. In other words, both bones at the joint increase in size as growth proceeds. (*From* Enlow D, Hans M. *Essentials of facial growth.* W. B. Saunders; 1996.)

between the bones of the eye are growth sites and, in a similar fashion to the cranial sutures and other facial sutures, are important sites of compensatory growth.

The orbits expand primarily in response to the rapidly developing eyeballs. This is greatest between birth and 2 years of age and contributes to anterior and lateral displacement of the midface. The orbits complete approximately half of post-natal growth by age 2 years.[18,31] Adult dimensions are nearly attained by 7 years of age,[18] after which the rate slows considerably until maturity.[32] There is inferior and lateral expansion in this region secondary to changes in the anterior cranial fossa and maxilla associated with midface displacement. The intercanthal width reaches full maturation at age 8 years in females and 11 years in males and the biocular width at 13 years in females and 15 years in males.[11] Bony apposition on the orbital floor offsets the anteroinferior displacement of the whole maxilla and contributes to midface height.[23]

Midface/Nasomaxillary Complex

The midface is connected to the neurocranium by a circummaxillary suture system and the midline

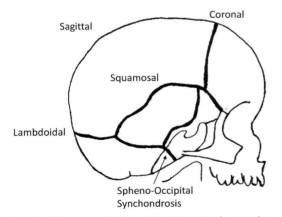

Fig. 6. Diagram of the calvarial sutural complex. Notice that peripheral sutures coalesce as they course inferiorly and medially, ending in the spheno-occipital synchondrosis.

by the nasal septum.[23] The nasal septum consists of the perpendicular plate of the ethmoid bone, septal cartilage, and vomer.[33] The nasal septum cartilage is continuous with the perpendicular plate of the ethmoid bone in the anterior cranial fossa at its caudal end and is firmly attached to the anterior nasal spine of the premaxilla through the septospinal ligament. The nasal septum cartilage is a growth center affecting vertical and sagittal growth of the nose and maxilla.[33–35] The majority of nasal growth occurs in 2 growth spurts, between 2 to 5 years of age and again at puberty.[35,36] Growth is usually completed by age 16 to 18 years in girls and 18 to 20 years in boys, although additional growth of the nasal septum may continue thereafter.

The maxilla moves downward and forward relative to the cranial base, accompanied by the orbits and nasal cavity, with each of these structures increasing in volume as they grow.[1] The zygomatic arches also grow laterally and are relocated in a posterior direction within the face. The zygomatic-arch length is 83% of adult length at 5 years of age. By 5 years of age, the bizygomatic width is 86% and the midfacial width is 89% of adult width.[15] The zygomatic bones provide midface width, cheek definition, and shape/definition to the lateral and inferior orbital borders.

The maxilla grows by (1) bony apposition at the circummaxillary and intermaxillary sutures compensatory to midfacial displacement and (2) surface remodeling (drift). Growth at the cranial base and nasal septum results in downward and forward displacement of the nasomaxillary complex followed by bony apposition at the circummaxillary and intermaxillary sutures[13,23] (**Fig. 7**). The facial aspect of the premaxillary–maxillary suture is partially ossified at birth, whereas the palatal region tends to close by age 6 years, although variability of complete suture obliteration with age has been reported.[37–39] An increase in maxillary width is achieved predominantly through growth of the midpalatal suture, with a smaller contribution from external remodeling. The midpalatal maxillary suture has been reported to close

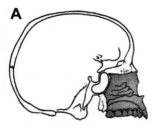

A

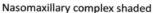

Nasomaxillary complex shaded

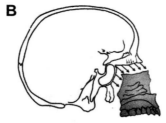

B

Displacement of complex

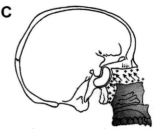

C

Compensatory bone growth at the sutures

Fig. 7. Maxillary growth. The whole maxillary region is displaced downward and forward away from the cranium. This then triggers new bone growth at the various sutural contact surfaces between the nasomaxillary complex and the cranial floor. (*From* Enlow D, Hans M. *Essentials of facial growth.* W. B. Saunders; 1996.)

between 15 and 19 years of age.[40] Sagittal growth of the maxilla continues until about 14 years of age in females and 16 years of age in males.[19]

A complex pattern of bone resorption and deposition occurs over the surface of the maxilla as it is displaced downward and forward within the face. Bone is deposited in the maxillary tuberosity region, contributing to an increase in length of the entire maxilla and creation of additional space for the developing dentition. Concomitantly, almost the entire anterior surface of the maxilla is an area of resorption. Growth and development of the maxilla parallels growth and pneumatization of the maxillary sinus.[41] Midfacial height increases due to the combined effects of inferior cortical drift and inferior displacement. The inferior translation of the maxilla is associated with bone resorption at the nasal floor (increasing the nasal cavity) and bony deposition along the hard palate.[6] The height of the midface is further increased by continued development of the dentition and alveolar bone. Vertical facial growth is the last dimension to be completed and continues into adulthood.

Mandible

The lower third of the face is composed of a single bone in the adult, the mandible. The mandible functions as a lever and a link for muscles involved in mastication, speech, and other oral functions. At birth, the right and left hemimandibles have not yet fused, the chin is rudimentary and retrusive, the gonial angle is obtuse, the ramus is short, both in absolute terms and in proportion to the corpus, and there is no appreciable alveolar bone. The developing primary teeth are discernible in their crypts on radiographs.

The mandible articulates at each glenoid fossa of the temporal bone in the middle cranial fossa.[13] As the whole mandible is displaced downward and forward relative to the cranial base, the condyle and ramus grow upward and backward (**Fig. 8**).

Although all aspects of the mandible increase substantially in size, the paramount posterior-superior growth vector of the mandible is achieved through the combined processes of endochondral ossification at the condyle and surface remodeling at the ascending ramus.[13]

The cartilage of the mandibular condyle provides movable articulation, endochondral bone growth, and regional adaptive growth. Its responsiveness to mechanical, functional, and hormonal stimuli set it apart from primary cartilaginous growth centers.[21,23] Therefore, the secondary cartilage of the condyle is more consistent with the concept of an adaptive, compensatory growth site.[42]

The mandible increases in size by a combination of 3 growth processes: endochondral bone growth at the condyle; surface remodeling throughout, particularly on the posterior ramus; and dental

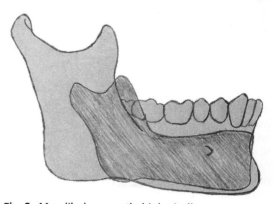

Fig. 8. Mandibular growth: biologically correct superimposition of the mandible registered on the inner table on the mandibular symphysis. The condyle and ramus elongate in a posterior and superior direction while the body of the mandible lengthens. There is little growth of the chin in the development of the mandible. (Adapted from Enlow D, Hans M. *Essentials of facial growth.* W. B. Saunders; 1996.)

eruption with development of alveolar bone.[13,43] Significant postnatal development is attributed to differential formation and modeling of bone along nearly the entire surface of the mandible, particularly along its superior and posterior aspects. The increase in ramus height and anteroposterior depth is achieved through resorption on the anterior surface of the ramus and greater deposition along the posterior surface of the ramus. At the same time, the corpus increases in length, providing the necessary space for development and eruption of the mandibular dentition. Associated with these changes in the absolute and relative sizes of the mandible are decreases in the gonial angle between the ramus and corpus.[23] The mandibular width increases by bony apposition along the buccal outer surface of the corpus and ramus and, to a lesser extent, resorption of bone occurs along the lingual, inner surfaces. Expansion of the mandible in the posterior direction via bone deposition along the posterior border of the ramus results in a longer and wider mandible.

At 7 years of age, bigonial width in males is 85% of adult width and in females 88% of adult width.[44] Growth in length and height of the mandible continues through the period of puberty. Height of the mandibular corpus depends in large part on growth of the alveolar bone. The mandible typically reaches adult size between 14 and 16 years in females and between 18 and 20 years in males.[16,17,19]

ORAL APPARATUS

The oral apparatus is composed of the dentition and the supporting structures within the maxilla and mandible. It is greatly influenced by the soft tissues such as the tongue and muscles of mastication.[23]

Teeth

The deciduous and permanent teeth are specialized organs of epithelial-mesenchymal origin. Normally, a complete set of primary teeth (20) have erupted by 2.5 to 3 years of age. The mixed dentition stage is heralded by eruption of the first permanent molars around 6 to 7 years of age. During the mixed dentition, both primary and permanent teeth are present. The mixed dentition stage is complete following the exfoliation of the last primary tooth. All permanent teeth except third molars (28 total in number) erupt by 12 to 13 years of age.

Alveolar Bone

Alveolar bone anchors the teeth and absorbs the stresses of mastication. Developing and maintaining alveolar bone depends on the presence of teeth. Prior to the eruption of the deciduous teeth, there is no appreciable alveolar bone. As the teeth erupt into functional occlusion, the alveolus proliferates in response to migration of the periodontal ligament. When a tooth is extracted, the alveolus at that site resorbs. If a tooth is surgically transposed or moved orthodontically into that site in the arch, alveolar bone will proliferate. In sum, the tooth is the functional matrix of the alveolus. Ankylosis arrests both dental eruption and alveolar bone formation in the affected area. Likewise, when a tooth is congenitally absent, the alveolar bone in that segment of the dental arch does not form (unless an adjacent tooth migrates into that space).

Appositional bone growth of the alveolar process occurs rapidly during the first 2 to 3 years to accommodate the deciduous teeth.[45] Dental arch width and perimeter change dramatically, especially during the transitions to the early mixed and permanent dentitions.[46] The teeth continue to migrate and erupt throughout childhood and adolescence, even after they have attained functional occlusion.[23] Teeth normally continue to erupt and form alveolar bone in synchrony with vertical growth. The posteruptive movements of teeth are directly related to the spaces created by growth displacements and movements of other teeth. The dentoalveolar compensation mechanism attempts to maintain a normal interarch occlusal relationship in the presence of variation in skeletal pattern.[47] Unlike teeth, dental implants are not capable of compensatory eruption or other physiologic movements.[48]

CLINICAL IMPLICATIONS
Anatomic and Physiologic Differences in the Pediatric Skeleton

Many age-related trends in pediatric facial trauma are explained by growth and development of the craniofacial skeleton. Soft-tissue injuries such as soft tissue avulsion, lacerations, and contusions[49] are more common than fractures in children, especially in younger children where the bones have a greater tendency to bend rather than break. Additionally, the facial nerve is in a more superficial position in the infant and young child, leading to greater chance of nerve damage in lateral facial soft-tissue injuries.[50]

A significant force of impact must be endured for the elastic pediatric craniofacial bones to fracture.[51] The pediatric facial skeleton has increased cancellous bone stock, larger buccal fat pads, decreased pneumatization of sinuses, buttressing unerupted teeth, and compliant sutures. These anatomic features allow the facial skeleton to absorb energy without fracturing and when fracture does occur, it more likely results in a greenstick or nondisplaced fracture[49,51,52] (**Table 2**).

The changing anatomy and physiology of a child affects facial fractures considerably. The ratio of cranium-to-facial skeleton, development of the paranasal sinuses, and stage of dentition all influence the incidence and fracture patterns observed. In addition, compared to adults, children exhibit greater osteogenic potential, faster healing rate, and capacity for significant dental compensation.[53]

Fracture Patterns and Locations

There is a higher incidence of cranial injuries in young children (less than 5 years of age) due to the large cranium-to-face ratio. In young children, a prominent forehead "protects" the later maturing lower face from trauma. The forehead during this period, therefore, is more exposed and prone to injury. Because of the lack of pneumatization of the frontal sinus before age 7 years, orbital roof fractures are more likely to occur.[54] In childhood, orbital roof injuries are considered fractures of the skull base. As such, intracranial injuries are frequently coincident.[51,54,55] Meanwhile, fractures of the orbital floor are relatively rare in children younger than 5 years. After age 7 years, there is an increased incidence in orbital floor fractures that coincides with growth of the maxilla and maxillary sinus pneumatization.[56–58] Children with orbital floor fractures are prone to entrapment[59] due to the elasticity of the pediatric orbital bone and potential for greenstick fracture.

Whereas cranio-orbital injuries are seen more in the very young, midface and lower face injuries occur more frequently in the older and adolescent child. As the child grows, the forward and downward projection of the face increases the incidence of midface and mandibular fractures.

Classical Le Fort midface fractures are rare in young children due to the presence of prominent buccal fat pads, immature sinus development, and buffering unerupted tooth buds.[52,60] Maxillary sinus expansion coincides with dental eruption during the mixed dentition, ages 6 to 12 years, and achieves full dimensions by puberty.[53] After age 6 years, maxillary fractures occur more frequently but the elasticity of the bone and mixed dentition may limit displacement. At age 12 years, which coincides with the permanent dentition and further expansion of the maxillary sinus, Le Fort midface type fractures become more common.[61] Similarly, zygomaticomaxillary complex fractures parallel the pneumatization of the maxillary sinus.

Midface fractures typically result from high energy impacts such as motor vehicle collisions and when present in young children, they are rarely isolated. There is a high incidence of associated neurocranial injuries because the force required to cause the maxillary fracture is sufficient to be transmitted to the cranial cavity.[62]

Likewise, nasal orbital ethmoid fractures (NOE) typically require high impact forces to the central nasal region. NOE fractures are rare compared to isolated nasal fractures,[63,64] which require less force to produce.[65] Nasal fractures are one of the most common pediatric facial fractures. As the nasal framework is more cartilaginous than bony, fractures of the cartilaginous septum are often found in children, whereas fractures of the bony nasal pyramid do not occur as frequently. Septal cartilage in children tends to buckle during trauma, making septal hematoma formation a more common finding than in adults.[36,66] Expansion of the hematoma separates the cartilage from the mucoperichondrium, obstructing blood flow to the nasal cartilage and causing pressure induced avascular necrosis of the nasal cartilage if left untreated.

The mandibular condyle is also a common site of fracture. Children younger than 5 years of age

Table 2
Summary overview of differences within the pediatric population

Infant/Child	Young Adolescent	Older Adolescent
Greenstick fracture	Fracture pattern variable	Fracture pattern may be adult-like
Small or absent sinuses	Developing sinuses	Mature sinuses
Developing tooth buds and challenging interdental fixation	Late mixed dentition/ permanent dentition	Permanent dentition
Bony healing occurs quickly		High energy trauma more frequent

are more likely to sustain intracapsular fractures and condylar neck fractures.[67] With increasing age, there is a shift toward subcondylar fractures and in adolescence angle and body fractures are more common.[36,67,68]

Growth Disturbance and Other Sequela

Trauma to growth centers (synchondroses, nasal septal cartilage), interruption of growth sites (sutures, periosteal absorption-resorption processes), damage to the mandibular condyle, and scar formation can disrupt normal facial growth and development. In addition, intraoperative soft tissue damage, periosteal stripping, and rigid fixation may affect the growing skeleton and developing dentition.[16,69] Interdental fixation is challenging in the mixed dentition.[53] Metal fixation systems carry real risk of injury to unerupted permanent tooth follicles and theoretical complications such as growth restriction (i.e., plate across suture lines). Bioresorbable plates and screws have been proposed as an alternative.[60] When internal bony fixation is necessary in younger patients, monocortical screws should be used and the hardware placed to avoid developing tooth buds.[52]

Generally, 3 main areas of growth may be affected: the orbital region, the nasomaxillary complex, and the condyle.[70] Dysmorphology may result from the initial trauma, the intervention, or a combination of both, during the growth years. Whether a growing child is initially managed nonoperatively or operatively, the patient and family should be made aware of the potential for aberrant growth resulting in asymmetries and occlusal discrepancies which may not become evident until adolescence.[53] Long-term follow-up is essential.

Orbital Fractures

Orbital roof fractures can be associated with dural disruption.[67] A very rare, delayed complication is a growing skull fracture that occurs secondary to a tear in the dura mater that coexists with the fracture, allowing intracranial content to herniate through it and widening of the skull defect. Following surgical correction, some children require a second operation to restore the axis of the orbit or correct orbital asymmetry.[67,71]

Fractures of the orbital region in very young children may also result in periorbital tissue atrophy and subsequent orbital volume loss. Because the development of the bony orbit is driven by the volumetric expansion of its intraorbital contents, namely the eyeball, in children with traumatic or disease-related loss of an eye, an implanted expander device may be used to sustain growth

of the orbit until skeletal maturity.[72,73] The cranium and orbits are about 90% of adult size by age 5 to 7 years. To avoid or minimize growth impedance, when possible, reconstructions are performed when growth is nearly complete.

Nasomaxillary Complex Fractures

Nasoseptal and midface trauma in children can result in progressive deformity of the nose and midface with both functional and esthetic consequences.[36,74] It has been suggested that the younger the child at the time of nasal septum destruction, the greater the long-term effects on midfacial growth.[74] Thus, "in the pediatric population, aggressive open septorhinoplasties are typically avoided until skeletal maturity, and early closed reductions are recommended."[67] Nonetheless, long-term follow-up studies of pediatric nasal fractures treated with closed reduction have reported that over half the patients have deformity of the external nose including bony and cartilage deviations, saddling, dorsum widening, and hump.[65,75,76] Grymer and colleagues[75] pointed out that 70% of the patients with nasal deformities at the time of their study had reported satisfactory results following the initial treatment by closed reduction indicating that improvements diminished with future nasal growth. Secondary corrections may still be needed at skeletal maturity.[67]

Severe midface fractures, both treated and untreated, have been shown to produce very high incidence of subsequent deformities.[67,77–79] These include maxillary hypoplasia, facial asymmetry, nasal airway obstruction, and malocclusion.[77–82] Complications are most pronounced in patients who sustained multiple facial fractures likely because of both injury burden and extensive surgery required for reconstruction.

Mandibular Condylar Fractures

Condylar fractures can result in retrognathia, facial asymmetry, mandibular midline deviation to the affected side, malocclusion, tooth loss or injury, temporomandibular joint dysfunction and/or degeneration, limited mouth opening, and bony ankylosis.[4,67,83–88] An opposing maxillary occlusal cant may also be observed.[89] Several studies have reported less growth disturbances in young children less than 5 years of age due to high vascularity and regenerative capacity.[90–92] Demianczuk and colleagues[93] showed the greatest risk for significant growth disturbances was in the 4 to 7 year old and 8 to 11 year old groups, observing respectively that 24% and 16% of these children required corrective orthognathic surgery.

Patients with condylar fractures, whether unilateral or bilateral, may exhibit loss of posterior ramus height secondary to telescoping of the condylar fragment(s). Because children demonstrate remarkable bony remodeling, condylar fractures are frequently treated with closed reduction with a short period of maxillomandibular fixation as needed.[83,87,91] Zhu and colleagues[94] reported that in children aged 6 years and older, the condylar process remodeled incompletely. However, the remodeling of the glenoid fossa and increase in ramus height compensated for the hypotrophy of the condylar process on the fractured side. As children age, the ability to remodel and spontaneously heal is reduced. Mild malocclusions from minimally displaced fractures have the potential to resolve spontaneously with eruption of permanent dentition and through bony remodeling that occurs with growth and function.[67,69] Patients who sustain multiple fractures of the mandible are significantly more likely to have an adverse outcome that those with isolated mandibular fractures.[86] The mandible is one of the last bones to reach skeletal maturity and as such is vulnerable to growth and functional perturbations after injury to the condyles.

CONFLICTS OF INTEREST

The authors do not have any conflict of interests, financial or otherwise.

REFERENCES

1. Cobourne MT, DiBiase AT. Chap 3: Handbook of Orthodontics. Postnatal growth of the craniofacial region. 2nd edition. Edinburgh: Elsevier Health Sciences; 2016. p. 67–105.
2. Ranly DM. Craniofacial growth. Dent Clin North Am 2000;44(3):457–70.
3. Carlson DS. Evolving concepts of heredity and genetics in orthodontics. Am J Orthod Dentofacial Orthop 2015;148(6):922–38.
4. Rottgers SA, Decesare G, Chao M, et al. Outcomes in pediatric facial fractures: early follow-up in 177 children and classification scheme. J Craniofac Surg 2011;22(4):1260–5.
5. Moss ML, Skalak R, Dasgupta G, et al. Space, time, and space-time in craniofacial growth. Am J Orthod 1980;77(6):591–612.
6. Björk A, Skieller V. Growth of the maxilla in three dimensions as revealed radiographically by the implant method. Br J Orthod 1977;4(2):53–64.
7. Björk A, Skieller V. Facial development and tooth eruption. An implant study at the age of puberty. Am J Orthod 1972;62(4):339–83.
8. Bjork A. Facial growth in man, studied with the aid of metallic implants. Acta Odontol Scand 1955;13(1):9–34.
9. Fields HW. Craniofacial growth from infancy through adulthood. Background and clinical implications. Pediatr Clin North Am. Oct 1991;38(5):1053–88.
10. Farkas LG, Posnick JC, Hreczko TM. Anthropometric growth study of the head. Cleft Palate Craniofac J 1992;29(4):303–8.
11. Farkas LG, Posnick JC, Hreczko TM, et al. Growth patterns in the orbital region: a morphometric study. Cleft Palate Craniofac J 1992;29(4):315–8.
12. Farkas LG, Posnick JC, Hreczko TM. Growth patterns of the face: a morphometric study. Cleft Palate Craniofac J 1992;29(4):308–15.
13. Enlow D, Hans M. Essentials of facial growth. Philadelphia, PA: W. B. Saunders; 1996.
14. Costello BJ, Rivera RD, Shand J, et al. Growth and development considerations for craniomaxillofacial surgery. Oral Maxillofac Surg Clin North Am 2012;24(3):377–96.
15. Waitzman AA, Posnick JC, Armstrong DC, et al. Craniofacial skeletal measurements based on computed tomography: Part II. Normal values and growth trends. Cleft Palate Craniofac J 1992;29(2):118–28.
16. Wheeler J, Phillips J. Pediatric facial fractures and potential long-term growth disturbances. Craniomaxillofac Trauma Reconstr 2011;4(1):43–52.
17. Bhatia SN, Leighton BC. A manual of facial growth: a computer analysis of longitudinal cephalometric growth data. Oxford: Oxford University Press; 1993.
18. Berger AJ, Kahn D. Growth and development of the orbit. Oral Maxillofac Surg Clin North Am 2012;24(4):545–55.
19. Proffit W.R., Sarver D.M. and Jr H.W.F., Chap 2: Concepts of growth and development. Contemporary orthodontics, 4 edition, 2006, Elsevier, Philadelphia, PA.
20. Carlson DS. Theories of Craniofacial Growth in the Postgenomic Era. Semin Orthod 2005;11(4):172–83.
21. Baume LJ. Principles of cephalofacial development revealed by experimental biology. Am J Orthod 1961;47(12):881–901.
22. Meikle MC. The role of the condyle in the postnatal growth of the mandible. Am J Orthod 1973;64(1):50–62.
23. Carlson D. and Buschang P., Craniofacial Growth and Development: Developing a Perspective, In: LW G., RL V., KW V., et al., Orthodontics current principles and technique, 6 edition, 2017, Elsevier, chap 1. St. Louis
24. Buschang PH, Santos-Pinto A. Condylar growth and glenoid fossa displacement during childhood and adolescence. Am J Orthod Dentofacial Orthop 1998;113(4):437–42.
25. Agronin KJ, Kokich VG. Displacement of the glenoid fossa: a cephalometric evaluation of growth during

treatment. Am J Orthod Dentofacial Orthop 1987; 91(1):42–8.

26. Ohtsuki F, Mukherjee D, Lewis AB, et al. A factor analysis of cranial base and vault dimensions in children. Am J Phys Anthropol 1982;58(3):271–9.

27. Melsen B. Time and mode of closure of the spheno-occipital synchrondrosis determined on human autopsy material. Acta Anat 1972;83(1):112–8.

28. Pattisapu JV, Gegg CA, Olavarria G, et al. Craniosynostosis: diagnosis and surgical management. Atlas Oral Maxillofac Surg Clin North Am 2010;18(2): 77–91.

29. Morris C, Kushner GM, Tiwana PS. Facial skeletal trauma in the growing patient. Oral Maxillofac Surg Clin North Am 2012;24(3):351–64.

30. Ruengdit S, Troy Case D, Mahakkanukrauh P. Cranial suture closure as an age indicator: A review. Forensic Sci Int 2020;307:110111.

31. Escaravage GK Jr, Dutton JJ. Age-related changes in the pediatric human orbit on CT. Ophthalmic Plast Reconstr Surg 2013;29(3):150–6.

32. Smith EA, Halbach CS, Robertson AZ, et al. Orbital volume changes during growth and development in human children assessed using cone beam computed tomography. Head Face Med 2022; 18(1):8.

33. Kim JH, Jung DJ, Kim HS, et al. Analysis of the development of the nasal septum and measurement of the harvestable septal cartilage in koreans using three-dimensional facial bone computed tomography scanning. Arch Plast Surg 2014;41(2): 163–70.

34. Verwoerd CD, Verwoerd-Verhoef HL. Rhinosurgery in children: developmental and surgical aspects of the growing nose. Laryngo-Rhino-Otol 2010; 89(Suppl 1):S46–71. Rhinochirurgie bei Kindern: Entwicklungsphysiologische und chirurgische Aspekte der wachsenden Nase.

35. Kim SH, Han DG, Shim JS, et al. Clinical characteristics of adolescent nasal bone fractures. Arch Craniofac Surg 2022;23(1):29–33.

36. Wright RJ, Murakami CS, Ambro BT. Pediatric nasal injuries and management. Facial Plast Surg 2011; 27(5):483–90.

37. Nicol P, Elmaleh-Bergès M, Sadoine J, et al. Incidence and morphology of the incisive suture in CT scanning of young children and human fetuses. Surg Radiol Anat 2020;42(9):1057–62.

38. Behrents RG, Harris EF. The premaxillary-maxillary suture and orthodontic mechanotherapy. Am J Orthod Dentofacial Orthop 1991;99(1):1–6.

39. Trevizan M, Nelson Filho P, Franzolin SOB, et al. Premaxilla: up to which age it remains separated from the maxilla by a suture, how often it occurs in children and adults, and possible clinical and therapeutic implications: Study of 1,138 human skulls. Dental Press J Orthod 2018;23(6):16–29.

40. Persson M, Thilander B. Palatal suture closure in man from 15 to 35 years of age. Am J Orthod 1977;72(1):42–52.

41. Lorkiewicz-Muszynska D, Kociemba W, Rewekant A, et al. Development of the maxillary sinus from birth to age 18. Postnatal growth pattern. Int J Pediatr Otorhinolaryngol 2015;79(9):1393–400.

42. Voudouris JC, Woodside DG, Altuna G, et al. Condyle-fossa modifications and muscle interactions during Herbst treatment, Part 2. Results and conclusions. Am J Orthod Dentofacial Orthop 2003;124(1):13–29.

43. Björk A, Skieller V. Growth in width of the maxilla studied by the implant method. Scand J Plast Reconstr Surg 1974;8(1–2):26–33.

44. Lux CJ, Conradt C, Burden D, et al. Transverse development of the craniofacial skeleton and dentition between 7 and 15 years of age–a longitudinal postero-anterior cephalometric study. Eur J Orthod 2004;26(1):31–42.

45. Laowansiri U, Behrents RG, Araujo E, et al. Maxillary growth and maturation during infancy and early childhood. Angle Orthod. Jul 2013;83(4): 563–71.

46. Moorrees CF, Gron AM, Lebret LM, et al. Growth studies of the dentition: a review. Am J Orthod 1969;55(6):600–16.

47. Solow B. The dentoalveolar compensatory mechanism: background and clinical implications. Br J Orthod 1980;7(3):145–61.

48. Oesterle LJ, Cronin RJ Jr, Ranly DM. Maxillary implants and the growing patient. Int J Oral Maxillofac Implants 1993;8(4):377–87.

49. Ferreira P, Soares C, Amarante J. Facial Trauma. Pediatr Surg 2021;501–33. chap Chapter 133.

50. Kellman RM, Tatum SA. Pediatric craniomaxillofacial trauma. Facial Plast Surg Clin North Am 2014;22(4): 559–72.

51. Oppenheimer AJ, Monson LA, Buchman SR. Pediatric orbital fractures. Craniomaxillofac Trauma Reconstr 2013;6(1):9–20.

52. Andrew TW, Morbia R, Lorenz HP. Pediatric Facial Trauma. Clin Plast Surg 2019;46(2):239–47.

53. Maqusi S, Morris DE, Patel PK, et al. Complications of pediatric facial fractures. J Craniofac Surg 2012; 23(4):1023–7.

54. O-Lee TJ, Koltai PJ. Pediatric orbital roof fractures. Operat Tech Otolaryngol Head Neck Surg 2008; 19(2):98–107.

55. Gerbino G, Roccia F, Benech A, et al. Analysis of 158 frontal sinus fractures: current surgical management and complications. J Craniomaxillofac Surg 2000;28(3):133–9.

56. Broyles JM, Jones D, Bellamy J, et al. Pediatric Orbital Floor Fractures: Outcome Analysis of 72 Children with Orbital Floor Fractures. Plast Reconstr Surg 2015;136(4):822–8.

57. Guyot L, Lari N, Benso-Layoun C, et al. Orbital fractures in children. J Fr Ophtalmol 2011;34(4):265–74. Fractures de l'orbite de l'enfant.

58. Koltai PJ, Amjad I, Meyer D, et al. Orbital fractures in children. Arch Otolaryngol Head Neck Surg 1995; 121(12):1375–9.

59. Grant JH 3rd, Patrinely JR, Weiss AH, et al. Trapdoor fracture of the orbit in a pediatric population. Plast Reconstr Surg 2002;109(2):482–9 [discussion: 490-5].

60. Meier JD, Tollefson TT. Pediatric facial trauma. Curr Opin Otolaryngol Head Neck Surg 2008;16(6): 555–61.

61. Chandra SR, Zemplenyi KS. Issues in Pediatric Craniofacial Trauma. Facial Plast Surg Clin North Am 2017;25(4):581–91.

62. Koltai PJ, Rabkin D. Management of facial trauma in children. Pediatr Clin North Am 1996;43(6):1253–75.

63. Park SW, Choi J, Park HO, et al. Are gender differences in external noses caused by differences in nasal septal growth? J Cranio-Maxillo-Fac Surg 2014;42(7):1140–7.

64. Lopez J, Luck JD, Faateh M, et al. Pediatric Nasoorbitoethmoid Fractures: Cause, Classification, and Management. Plast Reconstr Surg 2019;143(1): 211–22.

65. Kopacheva-Barsova G, Arsova S. The Impact of the Nasal Trauma in Childhood on the Development of the Nose in Future. Open Access Maced J Med Sci 2016;4(3):413–9.

66. Johnson MD. Management of Pediatric Nasal Surgery (Rhinoplasty). Facial Plast Surg Clin North Am 2017;25(2):211–21.

67. Chao MT, Losee JE. Complications in pediatric facial fractures. Craniomaxillofac Trauma Reconstr 2009; 2(2):103–12.

68. Cleveland CN, Kelly A, DeGiovanni J, et al. Maxillofacial trauma in children: Association between age and mandibular fracture site. Am J Otolaryngo 2021;42(2):102874.

69. Lim RB, Hopper RA. Pediatric Facial Fractures. Semi Plast Surg 2021;35(4):284–91.

70. Miloro M, Ghali GE, Larsen PE, et al. *Peterson's principles of oral and maxillofacial surgery*. 4th edition. Switzerland: Springer International Publishing; 2022.

71. Amirjamshidi A, Abbassioun K, Sadeghi Tary A. Growing traumatic leptomeningeal cyst of the roof of the orbit presenting with unilateral exophthalmos. Surg Neurol. Aug 2000;54(2):178–81 [discussion: 181-2].

72. Tse DT, Abdulhafez M, Orozco MA, et al. Evaluation of an integrated orbital tissue expander in congenital anophthalmos: report of preliminary clinical experience. Am J Ophthalmol 2011;151(3): 470–82.e1.

73. Chojniak MM, Chojniak R, Testa ML, et al. Abnormal orbital growth in children submitted to enucleation for retinoblastoma treatment. J Pediatr Hematol Oncol 2012;34(3):e102–5.

74. Verwoerd CD, Verwoerd-Verhoef HL. Rhinosurgery in children: basic concepts. Facial Plast Surg 2007;23(4):219–30.

75. Grymer LF, Gutierrez C, Stoksted P. Nasal fractures in children: influence on the development of the nose. J Laryngol Otol 1985;99(8):735–9.

76. Dommerby H, Tos M. Nasal fractures in children–long-term results. ORL J Otorhinolaryngol Relat Spec 1985;47(5):272–7.

77. Davidson EH, Schuster L, Rottgers SA, et al. Severe Pediatric Midface Trauma: A Prospective Study of Growth and Development. J Craniofac Surg 2015; 26(5):1523–8.

78. Kao R, Campiti VJ, Rabbani CC, et al. Pediatric Midface Fractures: Outcomes and Complications of 218 Patients. Laryngoscope Investig Otolaryngol 2019; 4(6):597–601.

79. Precious DS, Delaire J, Hoffman CD. The effects of nasomaxillary injury on future facial growth. Oral Surg Oral Med Oral Pathol 1988;66(5): 525–30.

80. Ousterhout DK, Vargervik K. Maxillary hypoplasia secondary to midfacial trauma in childhood. Plast Reconstr Surg 1987;80(4):491–9.

81. Macmillan A, Lopez J, Luck JD, et al. How Do Le Fort-Type Fractures Present in a Pediatric Cohort? J Oral Maxillofac Surg 2018;76(5): 1044–54.

82. Aizenbud D, Morrill LR, Schendel SA. Midfacial trauma and facial growth: a longitudinal case study of monozygotic twins. Am J Orthod Dentofacial Orthop 2010;138(5):641–8.

83. Ghasemzadeh A, Mundinger GS, Swanson EW, et al. Treatment of Pediatric Condylar Fractures: A 20-Year Experience. Plast Reconstr Surg 2015; 136(6):1279–88.

84. Thorén H, Hallikainen D, Iizuka T, et al. Condylar process fractures in children: a follow-up study of fractures with total dislocation of the condyle from the glenoid fossa. J Oral Maxillofac Surg 2001;59(7): 768–73 [discussion: 773-4].

85. Lund K. Mandibular growth and remodelling processes after condylar fracture. A longitudinal roentgencephalometric study. Acta Odontol Scand Suppl 1974;32(64):3–117.

86. Smith DM, Bykowski MR, Cray JJ, et al. 215 mandible fractures in 120 children: demographics, treatment, outcomes, and early growth data. Plast Reconstr Surg 2013;131(6):1348–58.

87. Cooney M, O'Connell JE, Vesey JA, et al. Non-surgical management of paediatric and adolescent mandibular condyles: A retrospective review of 49 consecutive cases treated at a tertiary referral centre. J Craniomaxillofac Surg 2020;48(7): 666–71.

88. McGuirt WF, Salisbury PL 3rd. Mandibular fractures. Their effect on growth and dentition. Arch Otolaryngol Head Neck Surg 1987;113(3):257–61.

89. Vesnaver A. Dislocated pediatric condyle fractures - should conservative treatment always be the rule? J Cranio-Maxillo-Fac Surg 2020;48(10): 933–41.

90. Chang S, Yang Y, Liu Y, et al. How Does the Remodeling Capacity of Children Affect the Morphologic Changes of Fractured Mandibular Condylar Processes After Conservative Treatment? J Oral Maxillofac Surg 2018;76(6):1279 e1–e1279 e7.

91. Du C, Xu B, Zhu Y, et al. Radiographic evaluation in three dimensions of condylar fractures with closed treatment in children and adolescents. J Craniomaxillofac Surg 2021;49(9):830–6.

92. Sahm G, Witt E. Long-term results after childhood condylar fractures. A computer-tomographic study. Eur J Orthod 1989;11(2):154–60.

93. Demianczuk AN, Verchere C, Phillips JH. The effect on facial growth of pediatric mandibular fractures. J Craniofac Surg 1999;10(4):323–8.

94. Zhu YF, Zou Y, Wang SZ, et al. Three-dimensional evaluation of condylar morphology after closed treatment of unilateral intracapsular condylar fracture in children and adolescents. J Cranio-Maxillo-Fac Surg 2020;48(3):286–92.

Epidemiology and Etiology of Facial Injuries in Children

Jeffrey Quinn Taylor II, DMD, MD[a,b,]*, Elizabeth Hopkins, MD[c],
Robin Yang, DDS, MD[c], Shelly Abramowicz, DMD, MPH[a,b,d]

KEYWORDS

- Pediatric - Trauma - Facial - Surgery - Nonaccidental trauma

KEY POINTS

- Isolated soft tissue trauma is the most common type of facial injury in the pediatric population.
- Because of the resilience of the pediatric maxillofacial skeleton, a considerable amount of force is necessary to fracture bones. Therefore, children usually present with concomitant injuries.
- Most pediatric trauma is preventable.

OVERVIEW OF PEDIATRIC MAXILLOFACIAL TRAUMA

Pediatric trauma results in over 8 million ED visits and 11,000 deaths annually in the United States (US).[1] Traumatic unintentional injuries continue to be the leader in morbidity and mortality in pediatric and adolescent populations in the US.[2–4] More than 10% of all visits to pediatric emergency rooms have been estimated to be a result of injuries to the craniofacial skeleton.[5] Most pediatric facial injuries are a result of isolated trauma to soft tissues of craniofacial skeleton (ie, 34%–92% of all facial trauma in children). Only 10% to 15% of those injuries result in facial fractures. The elasticity of the pediatric craniofacial skeleton allows for natural protection of the face.[6–10] Because of this elasticity and resilience, majority of all facial fractures in the pediatric population present with concomitant injuries.[1,6] Pediatric facial fractures account for approximately 5% to 15% of all facial fractures in children.[11–14]

Pediatric craniofacial fractures are rare below the age of 5 years; incidence ranges from 0.6% to 1.4%.[11,14] Craniofacial fractures become more common as children get older.[11–14] This is likely due to the increase of various activities that the child and adolescence population began to engage in (eg, accidental injuries from falls, contact sports and motor vehicle accidents) and their associated risks. Because children under the age of 5 years are not likely to drive a car or participate in contact sports, the mechanisms of injury for facial fractures in this population are different. In this age group, etiology of craniofacial injuries raises concerns regarding nonaccidental injury and child abuse (with child abuse being less common but an important consideration).[8,11] Male individuals make up the majority of those who are involved in injuries.[5]

Facial injuries do not often pose a direct risk of mortality, though in some cases they may be fatal due to damage to the nearby airway, digestive, and central nervous system. In an analysis of data from over 61,000 pediatric patients with facial injuries from the National Trauma Data Bank, Hebballi and colleagues found that risk factors for in-hospital pediatric mortality included ages 5 to 17 years, severity of facial injury, insurance status, and mental health comorbidities.[15] Other studies

[a] Oral and Maxillofacial Surgery, Department of Surgery, Emory University School of Medicine, 1365 Clifton Road, NE, Building B, Suite 2300, Atlanta, GA 30322, USA; [b] Department of Surgery, Emory University School of Medicine, 1365 Clifton Road, NE, Building B, Suite 2300, Atlanta, GA 30322, USA; [c] Johns Hopkins Children's Center Specialists, 6420 Rockledge Drive, Suite 2300, Bethesda, MD 20817, USA; [d] Children's Healthcare of Atlanta, 2105 Uppergate Drive, Atlanta, GA 30307, USA
* Corresponding author. 1365 Clifton Road, Northeast, Building B, Suite 2300, Atlanta, GA 30322.
E-mail address: jeffrey.quinn.taylor.ii@emory.edu

Oral Maxillofacial Surg Clin N Am 35 (2023) 515–519
https://doi.org/10.1016/j.coms.2023.04.001

identified midface fractures as having a particularly high-risk of mortality, likely due to their association with concomitant traumatic brain injury and damage to nearby neurovasculature.[15,16]

SKELETAL MATURITY

Maturity of the craniofacial skeleton occurs around ages 14 to 16 in girls and 16 to 18 in boys.[17] The immature craniofacial skeleton has unique features that allow it to respond to trauma in different ways than that of the adult. Bones in children are less ossified and are more likely to bend (ie, greenstick fractures) rather than break. The mandible and maxilla in children are insulated from external forces by additional facial fat pads.[18] In adults, the facial skeleton acts as a crumple zone to help decrease trauma to the brain. In addition, sinuses protect the vital structures in craniofacial skeleton and continue to develop until they reach their full adult size during the teenage years. The only exception is the frontal sinus that continues to enlarge into the second decade of life.[19] Furthermore, children have a decreased ratio of facial to cranial volume, and thus less structures overall to absorb impact.

ETIOLOGY OF INJURIES

The most common etiologies for facial injuries in children and adolescence are as follows[5,6,11–14]

- Motor vehicle accidents (55.1%)
- Assault (14.5%)
- Accidental injuries (eg, blunt trauma from falls) (8.6%)
- Sports injuries
- Child abuse
- Penetrating injuries (eg, stab injuries, animal bites, etc.)

Age-related development should be considered when deciphering the etiology of facial injuries. This is paramount to arriving at the appropriate treatment for each situation. Accidental injuries and falls are more common in children below the age of 5 years (accounting for around 43% of all facial injuries in this age group).[5,6] For example, nonambulatory patients that suffer facial fractures require a skeletal survey and social work assistance for concern for child abuse. Another common example is the need for a rabies vaccination and/or antibiotics a patient that suffers a penetrating or an avulsion injury from an animal/human bite, or a foreign body. Based on the etiologies shown above, it is believed that most pediatric facial injuries and complications are preventable in nature. For example, up to date immunizations

in children and their pets can prevent post-trauma complications (eg, tetanus and rabies vaccines). An increase in supervision could reduce risky behavior by children. However, with the increased push in independence in children at younger ages and less supervision in the adolescence population, this leads to an increase in risk-taking behaviors which puts them at higher risk of injury.

Injury Sites and Patterns

The distribution of soft and hard tissue injuries to the craniofacial varies considerably with age as the facial skeleton becomes more pronounced and mineralized. Most of the elasticity of the craniofacial bones is lost by the age of 2 or 3 years of life.[20,21] Younger children, because of the larger size of the cranium, usually suffer more injuries to this area. This relationship shifts to the face and the mandible as they get older.[22–25] For example, midface fractures are less common in infants because of the high elasticity and lower percentage of the face covered by it. Midface fractures are more common as children become adolescents because of the decrease in elasticity and the increase in growth. Fractures in order of frequency have been represented by age group in **Table 1**, and facial growth is represented by **Fig. 1**.

Fig. 2 demonstrates the pattern of injuries that are represented in the pediatric population in mandible fractures. Facial injuries are generally age dependent in location. Younger children typically get injured in the cranio-orbital regions. Midface and lower facial injuries have a high incidence in adolescents. Treatment of these fractures in the pediatric population differs than in the adult population. Nonsurgical management (eg, closed treatment) is generally preferred: the pediatric facial

Table 1
Age and facial fractures in the order of incidence

	Infant	Child	Adolescent
Skull	1	2	5
Midface	5	5	3
Orbit	3	4	4
Nasal	4	3	2
Mandible	2	1	1

The following table represents commonality from 1 (being the most common) to 5 (being the least common).

From Horswell, B.B., Meara, D.J. (2022). Pediatric Facial Trauma. In: Miloro, M., Ghali, G.E., Larsen, P.E., Waite, P. (eds) Peterson's Principles of Oral and Maxillofacial Surgery. Springer, Cham.

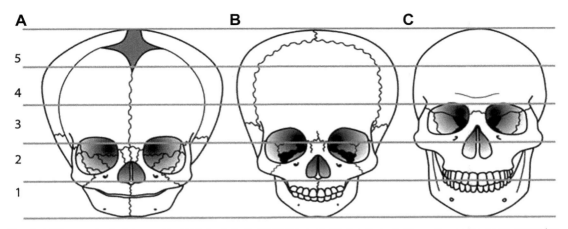

Fig. 1. Difference in facial growth. (*A*) infant skull, (*B*) Child skull, (*C*) Adult skull. (*From* Rengasamy Venugopalan, S., Allareddy, V. (2022). Craniofacial Growth and Development. In: Miloro, M., Ghali, G.E., Larsen, P.E., Waite, P. (eds) Peterson's Principles of Oral and Maxillofacial Surgery. Springer, Cham.)

skeleton demonstrates more rapid healing and has a greater potential for remodeling of displaced fractures than the adult facial skeleton.[26]

In the past, the propensity of a closed treatment may have been somewhat influenced by economic factors. Jenny and colleagues found that after implementation of the Affordable Care Act, significantly more children with facial fractures underwent open treatments. These patients also had significantly longer hospital stays and significantly increased hospital costs compared to before the Affordable Care Act (**Table 2**). Their data also show that, although overall the Affordable Care Act seems to have helped improve some of the racial disparities in treatment of facial fractures,

female and African American patients still had decreased likelihood of undergoing fracture reduction.[27]

It is important to note that facial trauma does not often occur in isolation. Facial fractures occurring along with injuries to other body systems are generally more severe, necessitating operative management.[28] Swanson and colleagues found a significant association between complications after mandible fractures (eg, malocclusion, facial asymmetry, hardware exposure, temporomandibular joint dysfunction) and the presence of cervical spine and skull base injuries. In fact, among the 116 pediatric mandible fracture patients in their study, over half presented with extramandibular injuries. Approximately 30% presented with skull fractures, 27% with midface fractures, and 17% with other intracranial injuries.[27]

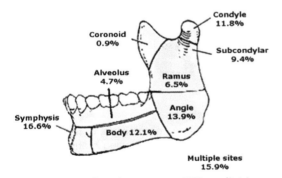

Fig. 2. Fracture location among 4169 pediatric patients with mandible fractures (age 0–18 years).[5] Fractures in the condyle and subcondylar region decrease as growth and development continues and body and angle fractures increase with age.[1] (*From* Imahara SD, Hopper RA, Wang J, Rivara FP, Klein MB. Patterns and outcomes of pediatric facial fractures in the United States: a survey of the National Trauma Data Bank. J Am Coll Surg. 2008;207(5):710-716.)

Nonaccidental Trauma

Nonaccidental trauma causes significant physical and psychosocial morbidity in children. Most abuse occur in children under the age of 5 years.[20,28] In the US, abusive head trauma is the leading cause of mortality among nonaccidental trauma in this population.[29] It is extremely important for the maxillofacial surgeon to recognize patterns and know when to seek additional help. A study done by Wasicek and colleagues in 2020 looked in the national trauma databank for an 8 year period for pediatric patients who were under the age of 5 years and suffered facial fractures.[30] They found that out of the 9741 patients included in their study 2% of those patients suffered injuries from nonaccidental trauma. This study also found that patients were more likely to

Table 2
Bivariate analysis of clinical presentation and management of pediatric mandible fractures pre- and post-implementation of the Affordable Care Act (ACA)

	Overall (%)	Pre-ACA (%)	Post-ACA (%)	*P*-value
Mean total no. of facial fracture diagnoses	1.50 ± 0.77	1.52 ± 0.77	1.32 ± 0.68	<0.001[a]
Reduction during hospital stay	40,059 (48.6)	37,024 (49)	3036 (44.4)	<0.001[a]
Open reduction during hospital stay	24,996 (30.3)	22,733 (30.1)	2263 (33.1)	<0.001[a]
Mean total no. of diagnoses	6.38 ± 4.51	6.0.5 ± 4.1	9.99 ± 6.74	<0.001[a]
Mean total no. of procedures during hospitalization	3.19 ± 3.30	3.12 ± 3.23	3.96 ± 3.98	<0.001[a]
Mortality rate	1743 (2.1)	1582 (2.1)	160 (2.3)	0.172
Mean length of stay	5.13 ± 5.13	5.03 ± 8.26	6.33 ± 9.94	<0.001[a]
Mean hospital charge	$54,135 ± $97,283	$48,612 ± $86,489	$114,452 ± $164,797	<0.001[a]

[a] Statistically significant comparison of pre- and post-ACA (*P*-value below 0.05 was considered to be statistically significant).[1]

From Jenny HE, Yesantharao P, Redett RJ, Yang R. National Trends in Pediatric Facial Fractures: The Impact of Health Care Policy. Plast Reconstr Surg. 2021;147(2):432-441.

sustain mandible fractures when there were non-accidental injuries and less likely to sustain maxilla or orbital fractures (which were more common in purely accidental injuries). Condyle fractures were the most common in the nonaccidental trauma.[30] However, the leading predictor at this time for the suspicion of nonaccidental injury is clinical context and should be carefully considered with any pediatric trauma case. Because the management of these fractures in the pediatric population differs from adults, it is important to think about the origin and mechanism of injury.

Pediatric facial fractures are associated with a significant health care burden, economic costs, and an increase in patient morbidity and mortality.[31] Reasons for this include both the presence of other injuries, particularly to the head and chest, and the fact that trauma to the facial skeleton can disrupt otherwise normal patterns of facial growth.[5]

SUMMARY

Injury to the growing pediatric craniofacial, maxillofacial, dental, and soft tissues can be vastly different than that of a skeletally mature patient. The management and treatment protocols should be customized toward the patient's developmental age and/or functional disturbances. Although the incidence of pediatric trauma is high, management can often be minimally invasive. Surgeons must balance intervention with the ability for monitoring skeleton development and management of growth abnormalities during and after skeletal maturity.

CLINICS CARE POINTS

- Majority of craniofacial fractures in patients younger than 5 years old are typically nondisplaced. Closed treatment is preferred treatment.
- When children are found to have craniofacial fractures without a clear etiology, nonaccidental trauma should be investigated. A skeletal survey and social work consult should be considered.

DISCLOSURE

The authors have no commercial or financial conflicts of interest in the following manuscript. The following manuscript has no funding associated with it.

REFERENCES

1. Andrew TW, Morbia R, Lorenz HP. Pediatric Facial Trauma. Clin Plast Surg 2019;46(2):239–47.
2. Cunningham RM, Walton MA, Carter PM. The Major Causes of Death in Children and Adolescents in the United States. N Engl J Med 2018;379(25):2468–75.

3. Borse N, Sleet DA. CDC Childhood Injury Report: Patterns of Unintentional Injuries Among 0- to 19-Year Olds in the United States, 2000–2006. Fam Community Health 2009;32(2):189.

4. Meier JD, Tollefson TT. Pediatric facial trauma. Curr Opin Otolaryngol Head Neck Surg 2008;16(6):555–61.

5. Imahara SD, Hopper RA, Wang J, et al. Patterns and Outcomes of Pediatric Facial Fractures in the United States: A Survey of the National Trauma Data Bank. J Am Coll Surg 2008;207(5):710–6.

6. Grunwaldt L, Smith DM, Zuckerbraun NS, et al. Pediatric Facial Fractures: Demographics, Injury Patterns, and Associated Injuries in 772 Consecutive Patients. Plast Reconstr Surg 2011;128(6):1263–71.

7. Zerfowski M, Bremerich A. Facial trauma in children and adolescents. Clin Oral Investig 1998;2(3):120–4.

8. Vyas RM, Dickinson BP, Wasson KL, et al. Pediatric Facial Fractures: Current National Incidence, Distribution, and Health Care Resource Use. J Craniofac Surg 2008;19(2):339–49.

9. Shaikh ZS, Worrall SF. Epidemiology of facial trauma in a sample of patients aged 1–18 years. Injury 2002;33(8):669–71.

10. Hogg NJV, Horswell BB. Soft tissue pediatric facial trauma: a review. J Can Dent Assoc 2006;72(6):549–52.

11. Cole P, Kaufman Y, Hollier LH. Managing the Pediatric Facial Fracture. Craniomaxillofacial Trauma Reconstr 2009;2(2):77–83.

12. Kaban LB. Diagnosis and treatment of fractures of the facial bones in children 1943–1993. J Oral Maxillofac Surg 1993;51(7):722–9.

13. Mulliken JB, Kaban LB, Murray JE. Management of facial fractures in children. Clin Plast Surg 1977;4(4):491–502.

14. Dodson TB, Kaban LB. California mandatory seat belt law: The effect of recent legislation on motor vehicle accident related maxillofacial injuries. J Oral Maxillofac Surg 1988;46(10):875–80.

15. Hebballi NB, Xie L, Kane AA, et al. Estimated prevalence of facial injury-related mortality in the United States pediatric population. Dent Traumatol 2022;27:12813.

16. Elzanie AS, Park KE, Irgebay Z, et al. Zygoma Fractures Are Associated With Increased Morbidity and Mortality in the Pediatric Population. J Craniofac Surg 2021;32(2):559–63.

17. Posnick JC, Kinard B. Orthognathic surgery. 2nd edition. St. Louis, MO: Elsevier, Inc.; 2022.

18. Chandra SR, Zemplenyi KS. Issues in Pediatric Craniofacial Trauma. Facial Plast Surg Clin N Am 2017;25(4):581–91.

19. Lee S, Fernandez J, Mirjalili SA, et al. Pediatric paranasal sinuses—Development, growth, pathology, & functional endoscopic sinus surgery. Clin Anat 2022;35(6):745–61.

20. Jenny C. Analysis of Missed Cases of Abusive Head Trauma. JAMA 1999;281(7):621.

21. Singh DJ, Bartlett SP. Pediatric craniofacial fractures: long-term consequences. Clin Plast Surg 2004;31(3):499–518.

22. Posnick JC, Wells M, Pron GE. Pediatric facial farctures: Evolving patterns of treatment. J Oral Maxillofac Surg 1993;51(8):836–44.

23. Haug RH, Foss J. Maxillofacial injuries in the pediatric patient. Oral Surg Oral Med Oral Pathol Oral Radiol Endodontology 2000;90(2):126–34.

24. McGraw-Wall B. Facial Fractures in Children. Facial Plast Surg 1990;7(03):198–205.

25. Morris C, Kushner GM, Tiwana PS. Facial Skeletal Trauma in the Growing Patient. Oral Maxillofac Surg Clin N Am 2012;24(3):351–64.

26. Swanson EW, Susarla SM, Ghasemzadeh A, et al. Application of the Mandible Injury Severity Score to Pediatric Mandibular Fractures. J Oral Maxillofac Surg 2015;73(7):1341–9.

27. Jenny HE, Yesantharao P, Redett RJ, et al. National Trends in Pediatric Facial Fractures: The Impact of Health Care Policy. Plast Reconstr Surg 2021;147(2):432–41.

28. Rosenfeld EH, Johnson B, Wesson DE, et al. Understanding non-accidental trauma in the United States: A national trauma databank study. J Pediatr Surg 2020;55(4):693–7.

29. Centers for Disease Control and Prevention. Preventing Abusive Head Trauma. Published online April 6, 2022. Available at: https://www.cdc.gov/violenceprevention/childabuseandneglect/Abusive-Head-Trauma.html.

30. Wasicek PJ, Gebran SG, Elegbede A, et al. Differences in Facial Fracture Patterns in Pediatric Nonaccidental Trauma. J Craniofac Surg 2020;31(4):956–9.

31. Yesantharao PS, Jenny HE, Lopez J, et al. The Impact of Payment Reform on Pediatric Craniofacial Fracture Care in Maryland. Craniomaxillofacial Trauma Reconstr 2021;14(4):308–16.

Intermaxillary Fixation in the Primary and Mixed Dentition

Jeffrey S. Marschall, DMD, MD, MS[a],*, Suzanne Barnes, DMD[b],
George M. Kushner, DMD, MD[b]

KEYWORDS

- Risdon cable • Arch bar • Maxillomandibular fixation • Intermaxillary fixation • Pediatric
- Primary dentition • Mixed dentition

KEY POINTS

- Do not use intermaxillary fixation screws in children because damage to the developing teeth is likely.
- Traditional arch bars may not be useful. Consider Risdon cable use, especially for those patients in the primary dentition.
- Use of elastics for maxillomandibular fixation is preferable over wires.
- Appreciate the key anatomic differences of the primary dentition.

INTRODUCTION

As society has progressed, so too have the mechanisms of trauma to the maxillofacial complex. As such, the management of craniomaxillofacial trauma has evolved gradually over time. Much of these changes were facilitated by the devastating injuries encountered during World War I and World War II. The studies of Kanzanjian, Converse, Gillies, and Millard are a testament to some of the great advances observed during this time.[1–4] The principles established by the aforementioned surgeons were further advanced by Rowe, Kiley, Curtis, Ivy, and Dingman in the midtwentieth century.[5–7] During this same relative time period, there was a tremendous contribution by Paul Tessier, who established the fundamental principles of surgical reconstruction of pediatric craniofacial deformity, most notably in Crouzon and Apert syndrome.[8] The common thread throughout the past 150 years of facial fracture treatment has been the understanding of the precise relationship of the teeth and how to recapitulate the preinjury occlusion. That is, if the surgeon places the teeth in their proper position, the bone generally follows. This same concept holds true for the management of pediatric mandible fractures. The definition of pediatric is somewhat variable, the focus of this article will be patients in the primary and mixed dentition, approximately aged 12 years and younger.

GENERAL CONSIDERATIONS
Anatomy of the Growing Mandible, Stages of Dentition, and Fracture Patterns

Although these general principles are discussed in detail by other articles in this issue, the discussion of intermaxillary fixation in children would not be complete without the mention of general anatomic and epidemiologic issues. During early development the thick periosteum and mandibular bone has a robust inherent osteogenic potential. This characteristic, along with the large medullary space and thin cortical walls of the mandible, yield much greater elasticity. This, in turn, results in a higher amount of greenstick fractures that are almost exclusively seen in pediatric patients.

a Department of Oral and Maxillofacial Surgery, University of Iowa Hospital and Clinics, 200 Hawkins Drive, Iowa City, IA 52242, USA; b Department of Oral and Maxillofacial Surgery, University of Louisville School of Dentistry, 501 South Preston Street, Louisville, KY 40202, USA
* Corresponding author.
E-mail address: jsmarschall@uiowa.edu

Oral Maxillofacial Surg Clin N Am 35 (2023) 521–527
https://doi.org/10.1016/j.coms.2023.04.002
1042-3699/23/Published by Elsevier Inc.

During the first few years of life, tooth buds make up a small percentage of the mass of the maxilla and mandible. However, as development occurs and the primary dentition and developing permanent dentition occupy the space of the mandible, the mandible is weakened, which facilitates fractures through these areas. Fundamental to understanding intermaxillary fixation is through a thorough understanding of the dentition. Pediatric mandible fractures can be divided into the stage of dentition of the patient; that is, fractures occurring during primary dentition, mixed dentition, or permanent dentition. The stage of dentition can greatly influence the modality to achieve intermaxillary fixation.

The tooth buds of the primary teeth are present as early as 12 weeks in utero.[9] The first teeth to erupt are usually the lower central incisors at 6 to 10 months of age. By 3 years of age, all 20 primary teeth are erupted. The pediatric dentition is characterized by short, bulbous crowns with different height of contours as compared with adult teeth. It is normal for the primary dentition to have spacing between each tooth, which allows for the eruption of the permanent dentition but also complicates traditional methods of intermaxillary fixation (ie, Erich Arch Bars, discussed later).

The mixed dentition begins at approximately 6 years of age with the eruption of the first permanent molar. The last primary tooth exfoliates at approximately 12 years of age. The simultaneous eruption of permanent teeth and exfoliation of primary teeth can lead to difficulty in establishing the proper occlusion and placement of interdental wires or arch bars. This combination can hinder mandibular fracture reduction for both open and closed treatment. As the child progresses into the teenage years and adolescence, surgical management of facial fractures and intermaxillary fixation techniques more closely resemble those of adults.

The mandibular fracture patterns seen in the pediatric population vary based on the stage of dentition.[10,11] The mandibular condyle is the most frequently fractured region of the pediatric mandible, generally ranging anywhere from 7% to 45%. This is followed closely by fractures of the parasymphysis, ranging 20% to 32% of fractures. Finally, mandibular angle fractures can range from 4.4% to 45%; however, this incident increases with the development of the third molar from the teenage years into early adulthood.[10–13] Potential treatment options for pediatric mandible fractures can range from observation, a short period of MMF and physical therapy, closed treatment with interdental wiring/arch bars and elastics, and open reduction and internal fixation. If anything other than observation is chosen, the surgeon must decide on the method of interdental and/or intermaxillary fixation.

METHODS OF INTERDENTAL AND INTERMAXILLARY FIXATION IN THE PRIMARY AND MIXED DENTITION

Methods of interdental and intermaxillary fixation in the primary and mixed dentition include Risdon cables, Erich arch bars, Ivy loops, sutures, and acrylic dental splints among other. Each of these treatment options has its own pros and cons. In addition, observation/nonsurgical management alone is often a prudent choice by the clinician (**Fig. 1**).

Direct Interdental Wiring

Direct interdental wiring is a simple, noninvasive way to aid in fracture reduction. In its simplest form, a bridle wire can be placed around the cervical margin of teeth adjacent to the mandible fracture to aid in reduction. In the pediatric patient, special care should be taken to not to avulse teeth. The wire can be left in place for 2 to 3 weeks, often in conjunction with arch bars or Risdon cables to help stabilize the fracture. The wire can be removed with ease in the office without the use of general anesthesia. Bridle wires are not a good option in children aged younger than 3 years. Patients in the primary and mixed dentition phases, roughly aged 3 to 12 years, the bridle wire method can be used but as stated earlier, the anchoring teeth must be stable.[14,15] The authors use this technique often, especially as a temporary stabilization method before definitive treatment in the operating room but generally in the late mixed dentition or permanent dentition.

Risdon Cables

Risdon cables are an ideal method to provide stabilization of the dentition and provide a mechanism to facilitate maxillomandibular fixation (**Fig. 2**).[16] The indications for the Risdon cable application include patients in the primary and mixed dentition that require stabilization of the dentoalveolar complex, a mechanism for elastics to hook on to, or an arch bar for maxillomandibular fixation.[1,2,16,17] The original description[16] by E. Fulton Risdon, Canada's first plastic surgeon, used a thick, 1-mm wire that was twisted around the last molar of the corresponding arch then braided to the anterior mandible parallel to the gingival margin. This was completed bilaterally, so that 2 wires were present on each arch. The 2 wires were twisted together at the midline, producing an "arch bar."

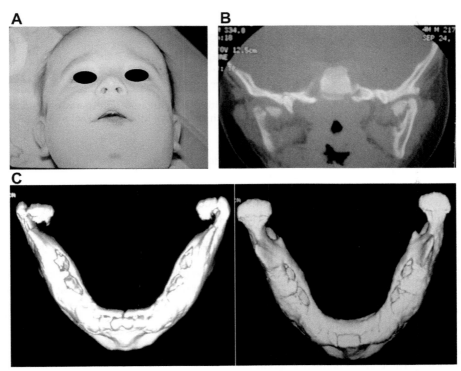

Fig. 1. Nonsurgical management of a bilateral mandibular condyle fracture in a 4-month-old child. (*A*) Facial photograph, note the chin and lower lip abrasions. (*B*) Coronal CT scan illustrating the bilateral fractures. (*C*) Three-dimension CT reconstruction of the initial injury (*left*) and of the fracture 9 weeks after injury (*right*), note the complete remodeling and healing of the fracture.

Modifications of the Risdon cable have kept the method contemporary and have made it easier to place, especially when operating solo. The preferred method that the authors use requires a 24-gauge stainless steel wire looped around the first molar and twisted from one side of the arch to the other. Next, circumdental wiring is completed around each tooth. If multiple surgeons are operating, this can be completed as one twists the arch wire, greatly increasing speed. This

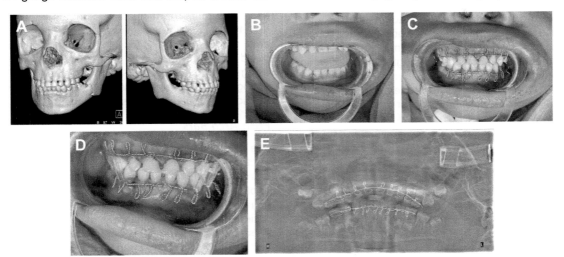

Fig. 2. A 5-year-old child with bilateral mandibular fractures treated with Risdon cables and elastics. (*A*) Three-dimension CT reconstruction illustrating the bilateral mandibular fractures, note the primary dentition. (*B*) Intraoral photograph with traumatic diastema and gingival laceration. (*C*) Intraoral photograph of Risdon cables in place. (*D*) Elastics used in place of stainless-steel wires for MMF. (*E*) Postoperative panoramic radiograph.

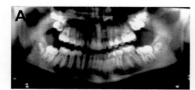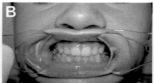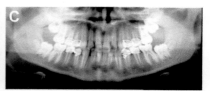

Fig. 3. Ivy loops utilized for short-term MMF in a child with a nondisplaced right parasymphysis fracture. (*A*) Initial panoramic radiograph. (*B*) Intraoral photograph with MMF established with Ivy loops. (*C*) Postoperative panoramic radiographic.

circumdental wires allow for elastic (preferred) or wiring to establish MMF. In addition to being a reliable method to obtain tight MMF, Risdon cables can also be used in dentoalveolar trauma.[18] The addition of autopolymerizing resin can be used to further stabilize the construct.[17]

Ivy Loops

Dr Robert H. Ivy was a professor of maxillofacial surgery at the University of Pennsylvania. His early method of maxillomandibular fixation has been used in adults and children for many years.[15,19,20] Ivy loops, also known as eyelet wires, are quick and inexpensive way to establish maxillomandibular fixation (**Fig. 3**). Three instruments are needed. The armamentarium includes a Backhaus towel clip, wire cutter, and wire driver along with 24-gauge stainless steel wire (for historical completeness, Ivy preferred brass ligature wires).[20] First, a 6-inch length wire is twisted around the tips of the towel clip forming a loop with 2 wire tails. After selecting the teeth to be wired, the ends of the eyelet wire are inserted from the buccal surface beneath the interproximal contact, if present, or the height of contour. One end of the wire is passed around the anterior tooth and the other end around the posterior tooth on the buccal aspect. One end of the wire (most commonly the anterior wire) is placed through the eyelet, which brings stability to the construct. The free ends of the wire are then twisted together. After twisting as tightly as possible, yet not breaking the wire, the wire is cut. This is repeated for the corresponding teeth in the opposite jaw. To establish maxillomandibular fixation, the upper and lower eyelets are connected by passing through a third wire bringing the jaws together while twisting.

This method has several advantages and disadvantages. First, the method is simple, inexpensive, and quick to apply. Considering the small amount of intraoral hardware, oral hygiene is generally improved. This can be an effective method in patients with areas of edentulous spans. The disadvantages, especially, related to pediatric mandibular fractures cannot be overstated. First, wires tend to loosen every few

days and will require tightening. This negates their use in long-term (2–4 weeks) maxillomandibular fixation, which we generally do not recommend in the pediatric patient. Furthermore, the design of the wires does not lend to elastic therapy. Finally, there is no continuous occlusal level control, which can be provided by an arch bar or Risdon cable. Therefore, use of Ivy loops in the primary and mixed dentition may be limited and primarily used for establishing maxillomandibular fixation for open reduction and internal fixation, or short periods of maxillomandibular fixation in nondisplaced fractures.

Sutures

The methods of maxillomandibular fixation described above have all used metallic constructs. An alternative to wiring methods or arch bars is the use of interdental silk sutures.[21] This method should be used in fractures that are not severely displaced or grossly mobile. Another advantage is that the wires can be cut with ease. This technique is completed with 0 silk ties. The suture is placed around the necks of the teeth and then tied in a knot. Three sutures can be placed in each quadrant. The tails are left long as they are tied together with the sutures in the opposite arch for intermaxillary fixation.[21] An advantage could be the perception by the patient and family using the terminology of "strings" versus "wires" during the informed consent process.[21] This method is not commonly used by the authors.

Erich Arch Bars

The closed management of a pediatric mandible fracture can occasionally be treated in a similar manner to an adult mandible fracture with the application of Erich arch bars. However, the placement is more technique sensitive for the pediatric patient (**Fig. 4**). The anatomy of primary teeth must be considered. The conical root anatomy and short clinical crowns can lead to an increased risk of iatrogenic avulsion of the primary tooth. In addition, for the patient in the mixed dentition, teeth that are still erupting may not have adequate clinical crown present to place a circumdental

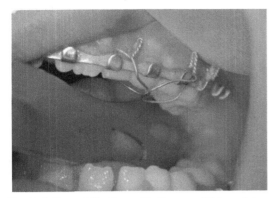

Fig. 4. Failure of fixation with the use of Eric arch bars in the primary dentition.

wire. If there are several teeth that have not appropriately erupted, this can lead to instability of the arch bar.

For the pediatric patient for whom placement of arch bars for closed management of a mandible fracture is deemed appropriate, the first step is to perform an appropriate history and physical of the patient. It is helpful to discuss with the patient's parent the presentation of the child's premorbid occlusion. If there was a malocclusion present

before the trauma, it is important for the patient and guardian to understand this will not be addressed during the surgery.

Once taken to the operating room, the patient is nasally intubated with a nasal Ring-Adair-Elwyn (RAE) endotracheal tube. The occlusion is evaluated, and it is determined if it will be feasible to obtain an ideal occlusion with closed reduction alone. Next, the Erich arch bar is cut to a length that will allow ligation of as many teeth in the arch as possible. Additionally, the arch bar is adjusted so that it fits passively against the teeth. The arch bar is placed at a level between the teeth and the gingiva, taking care to make sure it does not protrude into the gingiva. The arch bar is oriented so that the hooks face away from the occlusal surface of the given dental arch.

The Erich arch bar is fixated initially by placing a wire circumdentally around a premolar. With both ends of the wire extending to the buccal, the arch bar is placed again at the level of the CEJ of the teeth, and the wire is tightened in a clockwise direction. The wire is then cut and turned, again in a clockwise direction, to form a rosette that is directed away from the gingiva. This is continued along the length of the arch bar, working from one side to the opposite to ensure complete

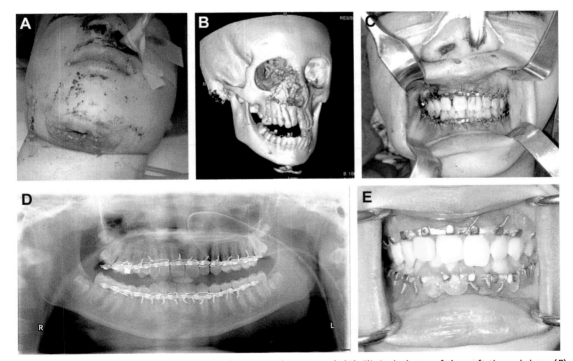

Fig. 5. A 10-year-old child who sustained a facial gunshot wound. (*A*) Clinical photo of the soft tissue injury. (*B*) Three-dimension CT reconstruction demonstrating the midfacial bony injury. (*C*) Intraoral photograph immediately after arch bar placement with elastics. (*D*) Postoperative panoramic radiograph. (*E*) Intraoral photograph taken at 3-weeks after injury.

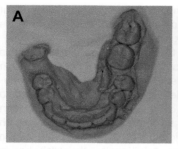
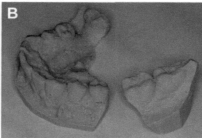
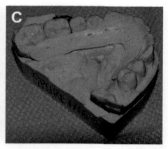

Fig. 6. Mandibular model used to fabricate acrylic lingual splint. (*A*) Initial cast. (*B*) Cast cut at the side of the fracture. (*C*) Cast fixated in a position that will facilitate fracture reduction with fabrication of lingual splint. Note the holes in the embrasure space for the placement of interdental wire ligatures.

adaptation of the arch bar against the dentition. At the conclusion of the placement of the Erich arch bar, it should be secure and immobile against the teeth and wires should not be cause for trauma to the soft tissue (**Fig. 5**).

After placement of the Erich arch bars on both the maxillary and mandibular arches, training elastics are placed to guide the patient into the appropriate occlusion. For the pediatric patient, healing often occurs at a faster rate than for the adult patient. As a result, if intermaxillary fixation is chosen with wires, a shorter time of MMF is often indicated.[1,15] Special consideration is indicated for the pediatric patient with a condylar fracture. If this child is immobilized for a significant amount of time, they tend to grow heterotopic bone and are at risk for ankylosis.

Postoperatively, patients are on a soft, nonchew diet for 4 to 6 weeks to allow for complete healing of the fracture. Jaw physiotherapy is encouraged, especially for a patient with a condylar fracture.

Lingual Splint

The use of a lingual splint can be very useful for the management of the pediatric mandible fracture (**Fig. 6**). This procedure is minimally invasive, can be advantageous in the patient with mixed dentition that may be otherwise challenging to obtain closed reduction and poses very little risk to the dentition.[22]

When considering a lingual splint for the treatment of a pediatric mandible fracture, it is helpful to obtain both maxillary and mandibular models. The mandibular model can be sectioned at the location of the fracture and then, using the maxillary model and an articulator, can be reapproximated to the patient's pretraumatic occlusion. The sections of the mandibular model are then glued together and stabilized. Once the mandibular model represents the patient's pretraumatic occlusion, it can be used to fabricate a lingual

splint using auto polymerizing acrylic. Holes are drilled in the lingual splint to allow for circumdental wiring that will maintain the splint in the proper position. The splint remains in place for 4 to 6 weeks and then is removed. Patients remain on a soft, nonchewing diet while the splint is in place.

SUMMARY

Clinicians must be acutely aware of the anatomic differences of the primary dentition and the challenges faced trying to recapitulate the preinjury occlusion in children. Clinicians should not use intermaxillary fixation screws, as damage to tooth buds will likely occur. Risdon cables are the authors preferred method, especially for patients in the primary dentition. Arch bars are an option, especially in the late mixed dentition. Use of elastics is preferred over tight MMF with wires.

CLINICS CARE POINTS

- Pay close attention the patients' stage of dentition because this will have a profound impact methodology of intermaxillary fixation.
- Consider Risdon cables in patients in the primary dentition.
- When possible, use elastics instead of wire to obtain maxillomandibular fixation.

REFERENCES

1. Kushner GM, Tiwana PS. Fractures of the growing mandible. Atlas Oral Maxillofac Surg Clin North Am 2009;17(1):81–91.
2. Morris C, Kushner GM, Tiwana PS. Facial skeletal trauma in the growing patient. Oral Maxillofac Surg Clin North Am 2012;24(3):351–64.

3. Coverse JM, Kazanjian VH. Surgical treatment of facial injuries. Baltimore (MD): Williams and Wilkins; 1949.

4. Gillies HaM DR. The principles and art of plastic surgery. Boston (MA): Little and Brown; 1957.

5. Thoma K. Traumatic surgeyr of the jaws. St. Louis (MO): The CV Mosby Co; 1942.

6. Ivy RHaC L. Fractures of the jaws. Philidelphia, Pennsylvania Lea and Febiger; 1945.

7. Dingman RaN P. Surgery of facial fractures. Philidelphia, Pennsylvania: WB Saunders; 1964.

8. Tessier P. [Total facial osteotomy. Crouzon's syndrome, Apert's syndrome: oxycephaly, scaphocephaly, turricephaly]. Ann Chir Plast 1967;12(4):273–86.

9. Tinanoff N. Development and developmental anomalies of the teeth. Philidelphia (PA): Saunders; 2016.

10. Siegel MB, Wetmore RF, Potsic WP, et al. Mandibular fractures in the pediatric patient. Arch Otolaryngol Head Neck Surg 1991;117(5):533–6.

11. Smith DM, Bykowski MR, Cray JJ, et al. 215 mandible fractures in 120 children: demographics, treatment, outcomes, and early growth data. Plast Reconstr Surg 2013;131(6):1348–58.

12. Glazer M, Joshua BZ, Woldenberg Y, et al. Mandibular fractures in children: analysis of 61 cases and review of the literature. Int J Pediatr Otorhinolaryngol 2011;75(1):62–4.

13. Posnick JC, Wells M, Pron GE. Pediatric facial fractures: evolving patterns of treatment. J Oral Maxillofac Surg 1993;51(8):836–44 [discussion: 844–5].

14. Schweinfurth JM, Koltai PJ. Pediatric mandibular fractures. Facial Plast Surg 1998;14(1):31–44.

15. Smartt JM Jr, Low DW, Bartlett SP. The pediatric mandible: II. Management of traumatic injury or fracture. Plast Reconstr Surg 2005;116(2):28e–41e.

16. Risdon F. The Treatment of Fractures of the Jaws. Can Med Assoc J 1929;20(3):260–2.

17. Madsen M, Tiwana PS, Alpert B. The use of risdon cables in pediatric maxillofacial trauma: a technique revisited. Craniomaxillofac Trauma Reconstr 2012;5(2):107–10.

18. Cho J, Sachs A, Cunningham LL Jr. Dental Trauma and Alveolar Fractures. Facial Plast Surg Clin North Am 2022;30(1):117–24.

19. Panesar K, Susarla SM. Mandibular Fractures: Diagnosis and Management. Semin Plast Surg 2021;35(4):238–49.

20. Blair VPal RH. Essentials of oral surgery. St Louis (MO): C.V. Mosby; 1923.

21. Farber SJ, Nguyen DC, Harvey AA, et al. An Alternative Method of Intermaxillary Fixation for Simple Pediatric Mandible Fractures. J Oral Maxillofac Surg 2016;74(3):582.e1-8.

22. Binahmed A, Sansalone C, Garbedian J, et al. The lingual splint: an often forgotten method for fixating pediatric mandibular fractures. J Can Dent Assoc 2007;73(6):521–4.

Rigid Fixation of the Pediatric Facial Skeleton

Kevin C. Lee, DDS, MD[a,b], Renée Reynolds, MD[c], Matthew J. Recker, MD[c], Michael R. Markiewicz, DDS, MPH, MD, FRCD(c)[a,*]

KEYWORDS

- Rigid fixation • Internal fixation • Resorbable hardware • Nonresorbable hardware
- Craniofacial growth

KEY POINTS

- Pediatric facial fractures do not often require internal fixation. Conservative management or closed reduction can be used for many situations.
- Internal fixation in children less than 10 years of age is complicated by the presence of reduced bone stock and permanent tooth buds.
- Nonresorbable hardware has superior mechanical properties; however, there are concerns associated with implant size, implant strength, translocation, and, less so, growth restriction.
- Resorbable hardware obviates elective removal and is a reasonable alternative to traditional titanium implants in non–load-bearing regions.

INTRODUCTION

Pediatric patients are distinct from adults. Children exhibit different facial fracture patterns; their bones are incompletely ossified; their dentition is constantly evolving; and their skeleton is actively growing. Furthermore, when considering pediatric care, the social concerns of both patients and their families may affect the timing and type of treatment rendered. Pediatric facial fractures are uncommon. Fortunately, the majority of these injuries are amenable to conservative management and do not require internal fixation. Due to ongoing growth considerations, many providers elect to avoid internal skeletal fixation in children whenever possible. Persistent plates and screws can potentially tether bony fragments and mechanically inhibit normal facial growth. It is important to recognize that hardware itself is not the sole culprit. Experiences borrowed from cleft surgery have demonstrated that there are multiple contributions to craniomaxillofacial growth restriction.[1]

Simple periosteal elevation disrupts the vascularity and the nutritional state of bone. Wound contracture and scar formation, which are part of normal healing, are well-described risk factors for subsequent bony hypoplasia. Furthermore, fractures or osteotomies can directly disrupt ossification centers. Even in the presence of these iatrogenic disturbances, growth is rarely arrested. As such, orthognathic surgery must be delayed until after adolescence to avoid skeletal relapse. It is difficult to parse out the contribution of each individual risk factor to growth restriction. This has led to uncertainty regarding the precise role that hardware fixation plays in altering pediatric craniofacial growth, with some arguing that internal fixation plays a minimal role in inhibiting normal bone formation.[2] Regardless, within many disciplines, there is hesitancy and preference against internal fixation in pediatric patients. The goal of this article is to present the principles of pediatric rigid fixation and to discuss the merits of nonresorbable and resorbable hardware options.

[a] Department of Oral and Maxillofacial Surgery, University at Buffalo, 3425 Main Street 112 Squire Hall, Buffalo, NY 14214, USA; [b] Department of Head & Neck/Plastic & Reconstructive Surgery, Roswell Park Comprehensive Cancer Center, Buffalo, NY 14203, USA; [c] Department of Neurosurgery, Jacobs School of Medicine and Biomedical Sciences, 818 Ellicott Street, Buffalo, NY 14203, USA
* Corresponding author.
E-mail address: mrm25@buffalo.edu

Oral Maxillofacial Surg Clin N Am 35 (2023) 529–541
https://doi.org/10.1016/j.coms.2023.04.003
1042-3699/23/© 2023 Elsevier Inc. All rights reserved.

PRINCIPLES OF RIGID FIXATION

Fracture immobilization is required to achieve bony union.[3] Primary bone healing occurs when precise anatomic reduction allows for direct lamellar contact. Once the defect is narrowed, osteogenic elements are then able to traverse the fracture line and restore continuity. If there is misalignment or movement across a fracture, the body will form a bony callus in an attempt to bridge and/or stabilize the bony segments (**Fig. 1**). Excessive gaps or movement can overwhelm the body's ability to heal secondarily and therefore increase the risk of fibrous or nonunion.

The concept of rigid fixation first originated in the orthopedic literature but was subsequently adapted for use in craniomaxillofacial surgery. Rigid fixation achieves complete immobility across a fracture such that there is no micromovement during function. In contrast, nonrigid fixation lacks sufficient strength to entirely prevent movement of bone fragments under function. Although rigid fixation is the preferred treatment strategy, the body can still achieve bony union with nonrigid fixation through secondary healing. Of note, when comparing fixation techniques, some surgeons will consider rigidity on a spectrum rather than as an all-or-none event. In this context, techniques that are better at reducing interfragmentary motion are considered to be "more rigid." The concept of rigid versus nonrigid fixation should not to be confused with the concept of load bearing and load sharing, the latter of which are properties inherent to the hardware that is used. With load-bearing fixation (reconstruction plate), the hardware absorbs all of the external force, whereas with load-sharing fixation (miniplate), the external force is distributed between both the hardware and the underlying bone. Load-bearing fixation is always rigid; however, load-sharing fixation may be either rigid or nonrigid depending on how it is applied.

Because the mandible is subject to both muscular and occlusal forces, the principles of rigid fixation are particularly important in the management of mandibular fractures. The upper and midface are not subject to the same functional loads, and therefore fixation strength poses less of a concern in those regions. Before the advent of modern skeletal fixation, closed reduction with maxillomandibular fixation (MMF) was the mainstay of treatment of mandible fractures. When situations were not amenable to MMF, external pins were used for rigid stabilization. Intraosseous wiring was helpful for aligning and reducing the bony segments; however, this technique was only semi-rigid and lacked sufficient strength to be used by itself in the mandible. Despite these and other early efforts at internal fixation, the end result always lacked sufficient rigidity. MMF was therefore still required as an adjunct to immobilize the fracture and eliminate masticatory forces. The first attempts at plate and screw fixation were met with high rates of failure because surgeons at the time did not respect the biomechanics of the mandible. In 1978, Maxime Champy published his ideal zones of osteosyntheses for load-sharing fixation in the dentate mandible.[4–6] Champy's techniques improved treatment success by optimizing areas of compression and tension to ensure adequate rigidity across the fracture line. A Champy-style plate for mandibular angle fractures is an example of "nonrigid" or "semirigid" fixation (**Fig. 2**) that functions with success because it respects the mandibular lines of osteosynthesis (**Fig. 3**).[4–6] Ellis subsequently expanded on Champy's work and proposed his own decision algorithm for managing non–condylar mandible fractures that incorporated both closed and open reduction.[7] This algorithm can be applied to pediatric fractures as well.

Pediatric craniomaxillofacial fractures are subject to the same treatment principles as adult fractures. Namely, the mandible preserves its role as a load-bearing bone, and therefore, any treatment

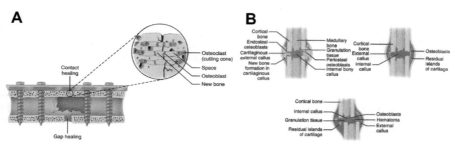

Fig. 1. Bone healing can occur (*A*) primarily when bone segments are in direct contact with no interfragmentary mobility or (*B*) secondarily through callus formation. (*From* Markiewicz MR, Engelstad M. Chapter 73: Principles and Biomechanics of Rigid Fixation of the Mandible. In: Tiwana PS. *Atlas of Oral and Maxillofacial Surgery.* 2nd ed. Elsevier; 2023:805-815.)

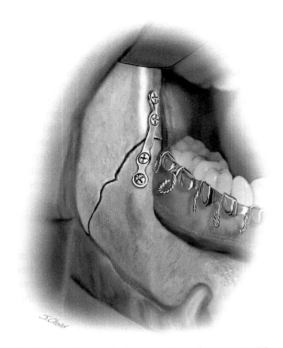

Fig. 2. The Champy technique allows for semirigid fixation of mandibular angle fractures using a miniplate with monocortical screw placement. (*From* Markiewicz MR, Engelstad M. Chapter 73: Principles and Biomechanics of Rigid Fixation of the Mandible. In: Tiwana PS. *Atlas of Oral and Maxillofacial Surgery.* 2nd ed. Elsevier; 2023:805-815.)

should incorporate the aforementioned fixation guidelines. Children do have the benefit of improved osteogenic capacity, and therefore, they can tolerate shorter durations of MMF. In

fact, prolonged MMF and temporomandibular joint disuse are contraindicated because they increased the risk of ankylosis. Their superior wound healing abilities and tendency to "greenstick fracture" also present a larger opportunity for conservative management. The designation of plates as either load bearing or load sharing by manufacturers is based on the ability to resist forces applied by the adult mandible. Children have lower peak bite forces, which places less demand on the hardware. As such, plates designed to be load sharing in adults may provide sufficient strength to achieve load-bearing fixation in a child. There is also a decreased need to obtain completely rigid internal fixation in children because dental splints and other external adjuncts are often used in combination to stabilize the fracture. The effectiveness of semirigid internal fixation for pediatric patients also opens the possibility of using resorbable materials not only in the upper midface but also in the mandible.

PEDIATRIC ANATOMIC CONSIDERATIONS

Pediatric proportions exhibit a larger cranium to face ratio (8:1) than that of adults (2.5:1).[8] (**Fig. 4**). As a result, the face is relatively protected from trauma at the expense of the cranium. Pneumatized sinuses and unerupted tooth buds compromise the structural integrity of the facial skeleton.[9,10] Stereotyped patterns of injury occur based on the stage of development and the location of these breakage points.[10–12] Midface fractures are extremely uncommon in children aged younger than 6 years because of the recessed bony anatomy, thicker subcutaneous fat pads,

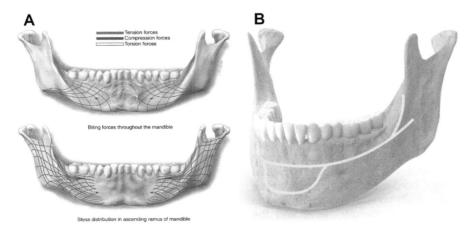

Fig. 3. (*A*) Each component of the mandible experiences various types of force during function. (*B*) The zones of osteosynthesis correspond to areas of fixation that stabilize the mandible against these forces and permit a favorable stress pattern. (*From* Markiewicz MR, Engelstad M. Chapter 73: Principles and Biomechanics of Rigid Fixation of the Mandible. In: Tiwana PS. *Atlas of Oral and Maxillofacial Surgery.* 2nd ed. Elsevier; 2023:805-815 (Figure 3A).)

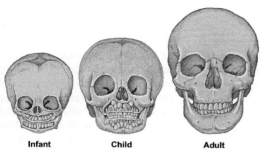

Fig. 4. The changing proportions of the craniomaxillofacial skeleton at various stages of development. (*Courtesy of* Paul Dressel, MD, Buffalo, NY; and Reprinted with permission from: Costello BJ, Rivera RD, Shand J, Mooney M. Growth and development considerations for craniomaxillofacial surgery. Oral Maxillofac Surg Clin North Am. 2012 Aug;24(3):377-96.)

and clinical irrelevance of the paranasal sinuses. The mature paranasal sinuses allow the face to absorb and dissipate forces away from the skull base.[12] The maxillary and ethmoid sinuses are present at birth and complete development sooner than the frontal and sphenoid sinuses that form postnatally. Once the maxillary sinus reaches a meaningful size, around the age of 7 years, the risk of orbital roof injury decreases and the risk of orbital floor injury increases proportionally with the extent of pneumatization. The pediatric mandible occupies a more vulnerable position in the facial skeleton than the midface and is most susceptible to fracturing at the condylar and the parasymphyseal regions.[12,13] The developing permanent mandibular canine creates a unique stress point that disappears once dental eruption and bone substitution are completed.[14]

The distinct anatomy of children also poses unique considerations for internal fixation. Most anatomic differences converge by 10 years of age, after which point many surgeons will manage both pediatric and adult patients in a more uniform fashion.[4,8] Until the eruption of the permanent second molars at 13 years, tooth buds occupy much of the intercortical volume within the mandibular body and symphysis. Even with grossly displaced fractures, bicortical fixation is generally unnecessary and relatively contraindicated during primary and mixed dentition (**Fig. 5**). Any internal fixation during this stage of development should be placed along the inferior border so that the screws are housed entirely within cortical bone. This avoids damage to the inferior alveolar nerve and the developing dentition. The pediatric maxilla is short and retruded, and before 6 years of age, much of the maxillary volume is similarly occupied by the permanent tooth buds. These maxillary tooth

buds may be at risk when attempting to plate the zygomaticomaxillary (ZMC) buttress for the rare pediatric zygomatic complex fracture. In such instances, Kaban and colleagues have justified using 1-point of fixation at the zygomaticofrontal suture because of the shorter lever arm generated by the smaller zygoma.[15] Every effort should be made to ensure that any internal fixation does not traverse suture lines or the mandibular midline.[16] Multiple animal studies have demonstrated that rigid fixation across active sutures in both the skull and the face mimics premature fusion and does significantly restrict growth potential.[17,18]

NO FIXATION

As previously stated, pediatric facial fractures do not often require open reduction or fixation. Their osteogenic potential and lack of bite force allows children to naturally recover from fractures that would not normally heal on their own in adults without surgery. It is important to recognize that a nonsurgical approach is distinct from "no management" or "no follow-up." In fact, the growing child benefits from closer follow-up than the skeletally mature adult. Pediatric condylar or subcondylar fractures are prime examples of injuries that are treated nonsurgically but require longitudinal observation (**Figs. 6** and **7**). Ideally, regular surveillance is performed by a multidisciplinary team that includes an oral and maxillofacial surgeon, a pediatric dentist, and an orthodontist. The growth of the mandible and midface should be monitored and consideration should be given to early intervention with dentofacial orthopedics, occlusal equilibration, or orthodontics. Midterm and long-term follow-up may reveal the need for subsequent surgical intervention to address acquired dentofacial deformities such as open bite malocclusion or facial asymmetry.

The aforementioned characteristics of pediatric patients permit reduction and/or reconstruction without fixation in select situations. Orbital fractures with single-wall defects generally do not need fixation. The supraorbital roof fracture is an injury pattern that frequently occurs in children and is rarely seen in adults. It typically presents as a blow-in fracture of the orbital roof, and when surgery is indicated, simple manipulation and reduction of the segments is often sufficient (**Fig. 8**). Similarly, implants placed for the reconstruction of isolated orbital floor fractures, whether through a transconjunctival (**Fig. 9**) or a transantral approach (**Fig. 10**), do not usually require fixation. Finally, isolated dentoalveolar trauma that spares the remainder of the mandible does not usually

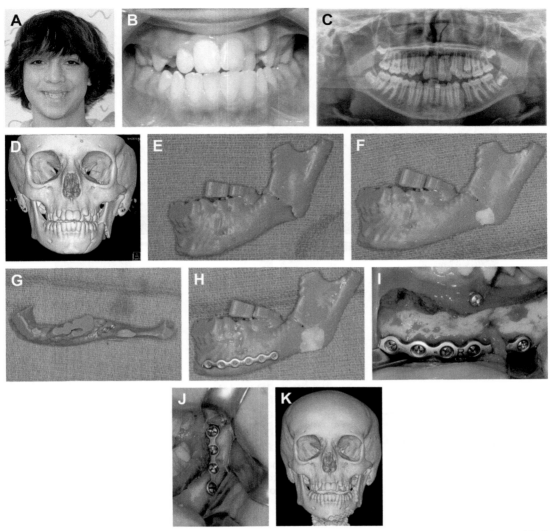

Fig. 5. Case of a 12-year-old patient who sustained a hockey puck injury to the face resulting in left mandibular symphysis and angle fractures. (*A, B*) Preinjury patient records obtained from orthodontist demonstrating a baseline Class 3 malocclusion. Left-sided mandible fractures demonstrated on (*C*) panoramic and (*D*) CT images. (*E*) In-house point of care printing of the left hemimandible using CT data. (*F*) Fractured segments separated and anatomically reduced. (*G, H*) Titanium plates prebent and adapted to the perfected model. (*I, J*) Excellent intraoperative fit of prebent plates confirmed without the need for additional adjustment. (*K*) Final immediate postoperative result.

require rigid fixation. Reduction into a semirigid dental splint provides sufficient stability for healing. In these situations, the senior author will often work in conjunction with a pediatric dental team to fabricate a 3-dimensionally printed occlusal splint for added rigidity (**Fig. 11**).

NONRESORBABLE FIXATION

The ideal implant has adequate strength to resist function, adequate stiffness to permit a thin profile, and adequate malleability to facilitate easy adaption.[19] Although early manufacturers experimented with stainless steel and Vitallium (cobalt-chromium-molybdenum) alloy implants, nearly all modern fixation systems use titanium because it has excellent mechanical properties, withstands corrosion, is biocompatible, and osseointegrates with bone. Compared with commercially available resorbable materials, titanium has superior resistance to both tensile and torsional forces.[20] Titanium implants are also more compact and less

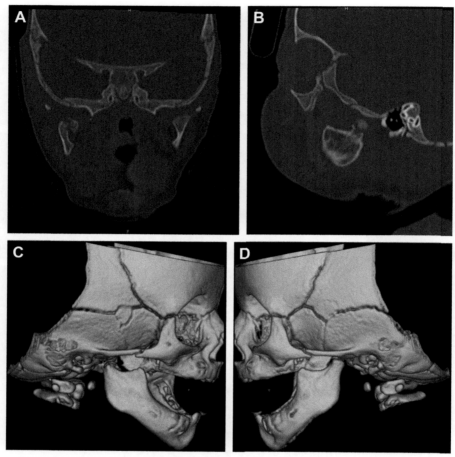

Fig. 6. Case of a condylar fracture in an infant that was managed with observation. CT of the face demonstrating medial displacement of the right condylar head on (*A*) coronal and (*B*) sagittal views. (*C, D*) Three-dimensional reconstruction of the CT scan demonstrating the loss of vertical mandibular height on the right compared with the left.

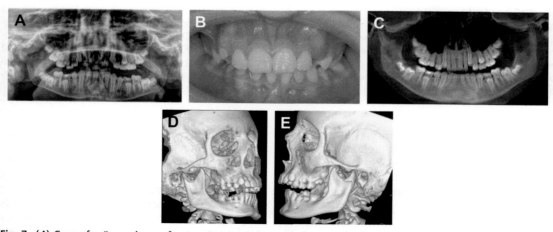

Fig. 7. (*A*) Case of a "guardsman fracture" pattern (mandibular symphysis with bilateral condylar necks) in a 7-year-old patient. (*B*) The patient presented 1 week following their injury with a stable occlusion, therefore the decision was made to manage them with observation. (*C–E*) Follow-up imaging at 5 weeks demonstrating up-righting of the displaced condyles and good secondary bone healing.

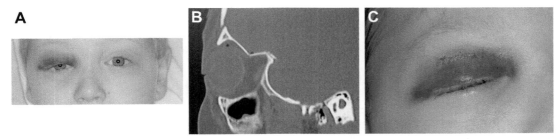

Fig. 8. Case of an 8-year-old patient who sustained an orbital roof blow-in fracture from a ball to face injury. (*A*) Preoperative photo demonstrating periorbital edema and ecchymoses with otherwise unremarkable ocular examination. (*B*) Imaging demonstrating displaced blow-in fracture pattern in the setting of a clinically absent frontal sinus and an incompletely developed maxillary sinus. (*C*) Fractured segments reduced without fixation using a periosteal elevator through an upper blepharoplasty approach.

palpable in the immediate postoperative phase. As in adults, the rigidity offered by nonresorbable fixation lowers the reliance on postoperative MMF. The ability of titanium hardware to protect the mandible from loading forces does raise the long-term concern of stress shielding, or disuse atrophy.[21] This effect is controversial and probably more of a concern with edentulous segments where there are no teeth to maintain the bone.

The inert quality of titanium permits the body to continue appositional growth around the implant. Unfortunately, this results in hardware translocation. Many surgeons who use nonresorbable plating in the growing child will perform a separate retrieval procedure between 2 and 3 months postoperatively once the implant is no longer serving its original purpose.[22] By doing this, the intent is to avoid issues associated with migration rather than address

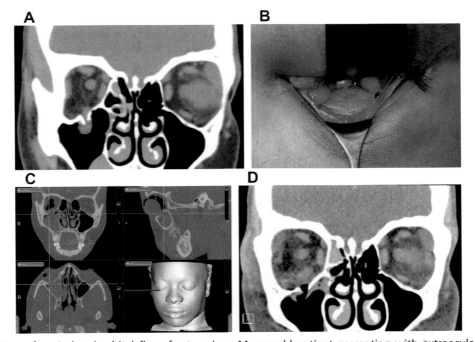

Fig. 9. Case of an isolated orbital floor fracture in a 14-year-old patient presenting with extraocular muscle entrapment. (*A*) CT coronal view demonstrating herniation of the inferior rectus into the right maxillary sinus, of note entrapment cannot be diagnosed radiographically and requires a clinical examination for confirmation. (*B*) Orbital floor reconstruction with a porous polyethylene implant placed through a transconjunctival approach without screw fixation. (*C*) Intraoperative navigation used to confirm the posterolateral seating of the orbital implant. (*D*) Postoperative imaging demonstrating reduced orbital contents. Porous polyethylene implants are radiolucent and therefore they are not visible on CT scans.

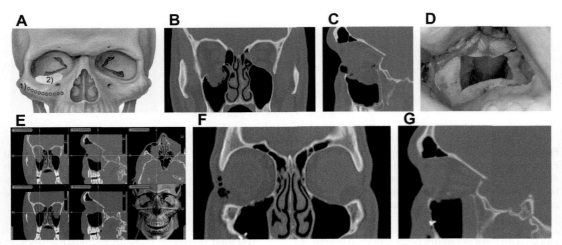

Fig. 10. Case of an isolated orbital floor fracture reconstructed through a transantral approach. (*A*) An antral window is removed from the anterior maxilla and replaced with fixation after the orbital floor implant is appropriately positioned. CT (*B*) coronal and (*C*) sagittal views demonstrating blow-out fracture of the right orbital floor. (*D*) Large maxillary antrostomy used to approach the orbit. (*E*) Intraoperative navigation used to ensure safe posterior dissection along the floor defect. (*F, G*) Postoperative imaging demonstrating reduced orbital contents and good form of the replaced anterior maxilla.

growth concerns because a second surgery itself could inflict additional scarring and growth restriction.[2,14] Furthermore, the fluid nature of bone remodeling argues against significant growth inhibition with nonresorbable hardware. When left in place, plates and screws can translocate into tooth buds or enter other body compartments, such as the intracranial space. Fortunately, there have been no documented cases of permanent brain injury from hardware migration. If the decision is made to leave the hardware in place, patients should be aware that approximately 8% of plates will ultimately require nonelective explantation due to pain or mobility.[2] Depending on the indication for removal, late retrieval of hardware can be quite difficult as the plates may be buried beneath a deep layer of healthy bone. Therefore, the removal of plates shortly after healing is recommended (**Fig. 12**). Hardware removal is usually no necessary in the skeletally mature patient (**Fig. 13**).

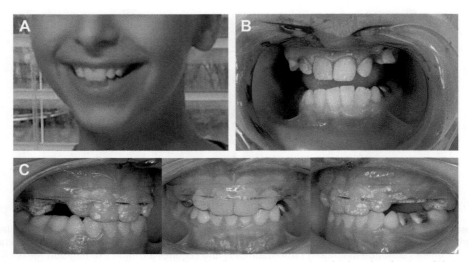

Fig. 11. Case of an isolated maxillary dentoalveolar fracture managed with closed reduction. (*A*) Preoperative photo demonstrating positive overjet. (*B*) Injury photo demonstrating edge-to-edge occlusion from palatal displacement of anterior maxillary dentition. (*C*) Postoperative result of patient after using both a semirigid wire and a custom in-house printed dental tray to splint and stabilize the maxillary dentition.

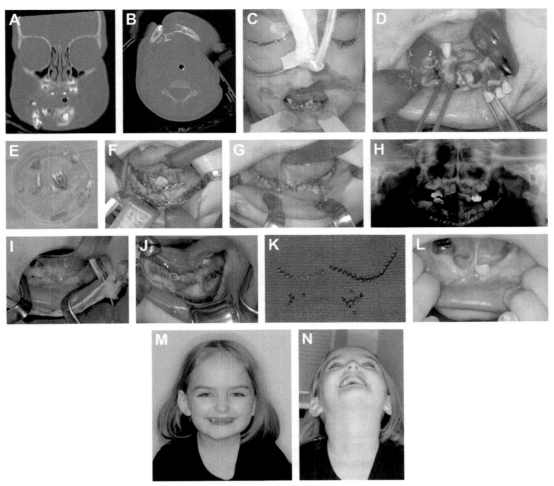

Fig. 12. Case of a 6-year-old patient who sustained a comminuted mandible fracture from an unrestrained motor vehicle accident. CT (*A*) coronal and (*B*) axial views demonstrating complex anterior mandible fracture with developing permanent dentition. (*C*) Clinical examination and (*D, E*) intraoperative findings significant for mobile dentition and multiple unsupported bone fragments. (*F, G*) Two load-sharing titanium miniplates used with monocortical screws to fixate the free-floating bone and provide rigid stabilization of the mandible. (*H*) Postoperative panoramic radiograph. Patient returned to the operating room 7 weeks later for the removal of the titanium hardware. (*I, J*) Exposure of the plates and screws was notable for bony overgrowth during the interval period. (*K*) Explanted hardware. (*L–N*) Three-month postoperative follow-up with good chin point symmetry and successful emergence of the permanent lateral incisor that was preserved in the zone of injury.

RESORBABLE FIXATION

The purpose of resorbable fixation is to selectively provide internal rigidity during the period of bony healing while avoiding the need for a second reentry procedure. Current resorbable materials are polymers of both polyglycolic acid (PGA) and polylactic acid (PLA). Both of these compounds are hydrolyzed into lactic acid. The lactic acid byproduct is then transported to the liver where it is metabolized into carbon dioxide and water. PGA degradation occurs more rapidly on the order of weeks to months, whereas PLA degradation takes years. Different manufacturers combine various proportions of PGA and PLA into their product so that they can obtain the desired degradation properties. Most commonly, resorbable hardware is designed to preserve its rigidity for up to 3 months and be completely resorbed by 1 to 2 years. Although titanium is radiopaque and prone to causing imaging artifact, resorbable fixation is radiolucent even if it persists beyond its intended duration.

The use of resorbable hardware is technique sensitive due to its less robust mechanical

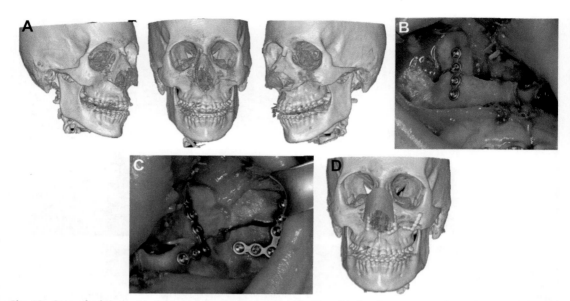

Fig. 13. Case of a bilateral Lefort II fractures with a left-sided hemi-Lefort I component in a 16-year-old patient. (*A*) Three-dimensional reconstruction of facial skeleton. (*B*, *C*) Transoral exposure of the hemi-Lefort I fracture with titanium miniplate fixation. (*D*) Postoperative imaging demonstrating reduced and fixated Lefort I fracture with closed reduction of the naso-orbito-ethmoid component of the Lefort II injury. Because of the patient's age and skeletal maturity, they were treated like an adult, and the hardware was not retrieved.

properties.[19] Titanium is malleable, and thinner plates can often be contoured in-situ. However, resorbable plates are brittle and need to be heated in warm water baths to permit adaptation. The weaker mechanical stability of PGA/PLA implants necessitates that they be manufactured to be broader and thicker than their titanium counterparts.[19] The larger footprint of resorbable fixation makes their use cumbersome (**Fig. 14**). Resorbable fixation is only intended for use in the cranium (**Fig. 15**) and midfacial skeleton (**Fig. 16**). It is not currently FDA-approved for isolated use in load-bearing situations such mandibular trauma, although some providers will combine resorbable fixation with dental splints and MMF to reduce the hardware strain.[23] As discussed previously, children have the benefit of a weaker bite force and smaller bones with shorter lever arms. Resorbable plates and screws seem to provide sufficient rigidity in most pediatric situations. Titanium fixation systems offer both self-drilling and self-tapping screw options to engage the bone and improve stability. Resorbable screws have poor torsional strength. As a result, they traditionally require both predrilling and pretapping before insertion. Even with proper site development, bioresorbable screws need to be carefully inserted because they are prone to fracturing during placement. In such instances, screw fracture is not catastrophic because the osteotomy can be

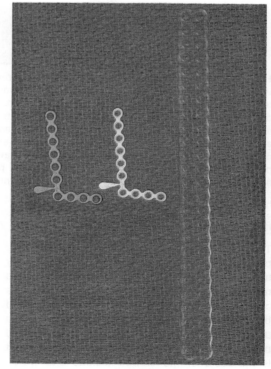

Fig. 14. Side-by-side comparison of titanium miniplates and resorbable hardware.

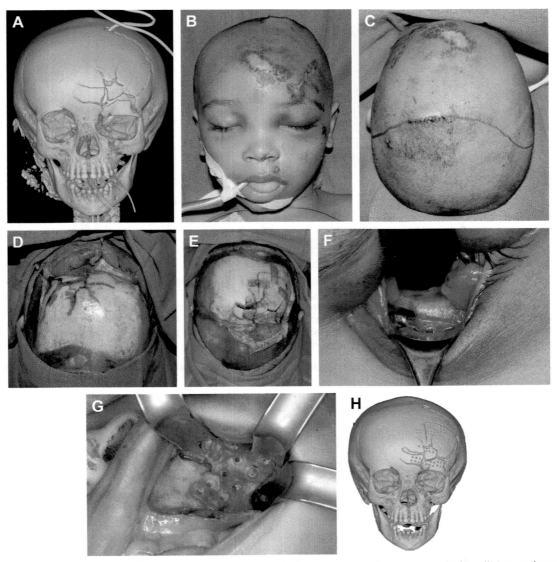

Fig. 15. Case of a 7-year-old patient who was an unrestrained passenger in a motor vehicle collision and sustained left-sided frontal bone and ZMC complex fractures. (*A, B*) Pattern of injury significant for orbital roof and floor components. Multiple scalp abrasions but no open laceration available for direct access to the upper and midface. (*C*) Planned bicoronal incision incorporating existing scalp laceration and extending short of the helical root. (*D*) Exposure of the comminuted frontal bone fracture. Note the clinical absence of the frontal sinus. Reduction and resorbable fixation of the (*E*) frontal bone, (*F*) infraorbital rim, and (*G*) ZMC buttress. (*H*) Final postoperative result. As with porous polyethylene, resorbable fixation seems radiolucent.

redrilled and retapped through the remnant shank.[23] Newer technologies have been developed to avoid resorbable screws altogether. Some manufacturers have incorporated systems that use ultrasonic energy to melt pin-shaped polymers into predrilled osteotomies so that the material engages the bony channels and improves retention while at the same time avoiding the pitfalls associated with torqueing of screws. Resorbable screws cannot be used bicortically, and this is generally not a limitation in pediatric mandibular trauma where bicortical fixation is avoided.

The complication rates seem to be equivalent between resorbable and nonresorbable fixation; however, few studies have directly compared both materials head-to-head.[22,24] Moreover, resorbable fixation is widely accepted to be safe for use in children.[24] The complications associated with titanium implants are well described and include extrusion/exposure, infection, hardware fatigue, palpability,

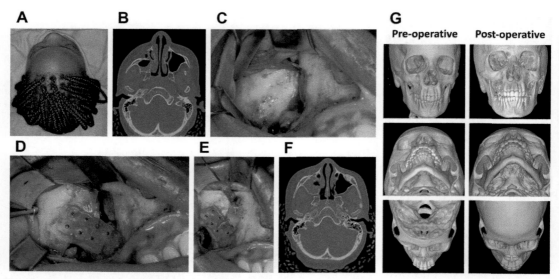

Fig. 16. Case of a right ZMC fracture in a 12-year-old patient. (*A*) Bird's eye view showing deprojection of the right malar eminence. (*B*) CT axial view verifying depressed ZMC fracture. The fracture (*C*) exposed through a transoral approach, (*D*) reduced with a Carroll-Girard T-bar screw, and fixated with resorbable plating. (*E*) Unsupported anterior maxillary bone fragment replaced and secured with bone sutures. (*F*) CT axial view of final postoperative result showing restored malar projection. (*G*) Comparison of preoperative and postoperative 3-dimensional renderings on frontal, worm's-eye view, and bird's-eye view.

and temperature sensitivity. Wound complications and hardware failure are also possible with resorbable implants; however, their transient nature may reduce the incidence of late complications. Many providers will account for the weaker mechanical properties of resorbable fixation during their treatment planning and elect to place patients into a short period of MMF.[23] This thoughtfulness probably accounts for the lack of difference in hardware-related failures when resorbable plates are used in the mandible.[22] A delayed foreign body reaction to microscopic PGA/PLA remnants can occur with bioresorbable fixation up to 2 years postoperatively.[24,25] This complication is seen in less than 5% of patients and typically presents as a palpable, fixed mass in the area of prior fixation. Larger volume implants are thought to be at higher risk for incomplete degradation, and these undigested remnants elicit a granulomatous inflammatory response. Fortunately, the offending fragments are fibrous encapsulated and usually able to be removed with a simple secondary procedure.[25] Finally, there is no convincing long-term evidence supporting the use of resorbable fixation for preserving growth potential. Provider preference and dogma dictate the choice of hardware because the decision is not currently limited by outcome data.

SUMMARY

Pediatric facial fractures are uncommon, and the majority is able to be managed with closed reduction or conservative therapy. Operating on the developing facial skeleton carries inherent risks of growth restriction and permanent injury to ossification centers and intrabony anatomy. Both resorbable (PGA/PLA) and nonresorbable (titanium) hardware are safe and appropriate in children. Resorbable implants are thought to reduce long-term complications but nonresorbable implants offer a more robust and rigid fixation. Most surgeons opt to retrieve nonresorbable hardware after 2 to 3 months of healing due to migration concerns. Growth restriction from internal fixation has multiple contributions. Properly placed hardware that respects natural suture lines is not thought to significantly inhibit growth. As materials science progresses, manufacturers can hopefully get closer to developing the ideal implant that combines the benefits of both fixation options.

CLINICS CARE POINTS

- Pediatric facial fractures do not often require internal fixation. Conservative management or closed reduction can be used for many situations.

- Internal fixation in children aged younger than 10 years is complicated by the presence of reduced bone stock and permanent tooth buds.

- Nonresorbable hardware has superior mechanical properties; however, there are concerns associated with implant size, implant strength, translocation, and, less so, growth restriction.
- Resorbable hardware obviates elective removal and is a reasonable alternative to traditional titanium implants in non–load-bearing regions.

REFERENCES

1. Von Den Hoff JW, Maltha JC, Kuijpers-Jagtman AM. Palatal Wound Healing:The Effects of Scarring on Growth. In: Berkowitz S, editor. Cleft Lip and palate. Berlin, Heidelberg: Springer Berlin Heidelberg; 2006. p. 301–13.
2. Berryhill WE, Rimell FL, Ness J, et al. Fate of rigid fixation in pediatric craniofacial surgery. Otolaryngology–head and neck surgery 1999;121(3): 269–73.
3. Jones JK, Van Sickels JE. Rigid fixation: a review of concepts and treatment of fractures. Oral Surg Oral Med Oral Pathol 1988;65(1):13–8.
4. Champy M, Loddé JP, Schmitt R, et al. Mandibular osteosynthesis by miniature screwed plates via a buccal approach. J Maxillofac Surg 1978;6(1): 14–21.
5. Michelet FX, Deymes J, Dessus B. Osteosynthesis with miniaturized screwed plates in maxillo-facial surgery. J Maxillofac Surg 1973;1(2):79–84.
6. Champy M, Lodde JP, Jaeger JH, et al. [Mandibular osteosynthesis according to the Michelet technic. I. Biomechanical bases]. Rev Stomatol Chir Maxillo-Faciale 1976;77(3):569–76.
7. Ellis E. An Algorithm for the Treatment of Noncondylar Mandibular Fractures. J Oral Maxillofac Surg 2014;72(5):939–49.
8. Meier JD, Tollefson TT. Pediatric facial trauma. Curr Opin Otolaryngol Head Neck Surg 2008;16(6): 555–61.
9. Totonchi A, Sweeney WM, Gosain AK. Distinguishing anatomic features of pediatric facial trauma. J Craniofac Surg 2012;23(3):793–8.
10. Kaban LB, Mulliken JB, Murray JE. Facial fractures in children: an analysis of 122 fractures in 109 patients. Plast Reconstr Surg 1977;59(1):15–20.
11. Imahara SD, Hopper RA, Wang J, et al. Patterns and outcomes of pediatric facial fractures in the United States: a survey of the National Trauma Data Bank. J Am Coll Surg 2008;207(5):710–6.
12. Posnick JC, Wells M, Pron GE. Pediatric facial fractures: evolving patterns of treatment. J Oral Maxillofac Surg 1993;51(8):836–44 [discussion: 44–5].
13. Hoppe IC, Kordahi AM, Paik AM, et al. Examination of life-threatening injuries in 431 pediatric facial fractures at a level 1 trauma center. J Craniofac Surg 2014;25(5):1825–8.
14. Goth S, Sawatari Y, Peleg M. Management of pediatric mandible fractures. J Craniofac Surg 2012;23(1): 47–56.
15. Mulliken JB, Kaban LB, Murray JE. Management of facial fractures in children. Clin Plast Surg 1977; 4(4):491–502.
16. Zimmermann CE, Troulis MJ, Kaban LB. Pediatric facial fractures: recent advances in prevention, diagnosis and management. Int J Oral Maxillofac Surg 2005;34(8):823–33.
17. Resnick JI, Kinney BM, Kawamoto HK Jr. The effect of rigid internal fixation on cranial growth. Ann Plast Surg 1990;25(5):372–4.
18. Southard TE, Franciscus RG, Fridrich KL, et al. Restricting facial bone growth with skeletal fixation: a preliminary study. Am J Orthod Dentofacial Orthop 2006;130(2):218–23.
19. Gilardino MS, Chen E, Bartlett SP. Choice of internal rigid fixation materials in the treatment of facial fractures. Craniomaxillofacial Trauma Reconstr 2009; 2(1):49–60.
20. Bos RR. Treatment of pediatric facial fractures: the case for metallic fixation. J Oral Maxillofac Surg 2005;63(3):382–4.
21. Pogrel MA. The Concept of Stress Shielding in Nonvascularized Bone Grafts of the Mandible-A Review of 2 Cases. J Oral Maxillofac Surg 2021;79(1):266. e1-.e5.
22. Pontell ME, Niklinska EB, Braun SA, et al. Resorbable Versus Titanium Rigid Fixation for Pediatric Mandibular Fractures: A Systematic Review, Institutional Experience and Comparative Analysis. Craniomaxillofacial Trauma Reconstr 2022;15(3): 189–200.
23. Laughlin RM, Block MS, Wilk R, et al. Resorbable plates for the fixation of mandibular fractures: a prospective study. J Oral Maxillofac Surg 2007;65(1): 89–96.
24. Lopez J, Siegel N, Reategui A, et al. Absorbable Fixation Devices for Pediatric Craniomaxillofacial Trauma: A Systematic Review of the Literature. Plast Reconstr Surg 2019;144(3):685–92.
25. Jeon HB, Kang DH, Gu JH, et al. Delayed Foreign Body Reaction Caused by Bioabsorbable Plates Used for Maxillofacial Fractures. Arch Plast Surg 2016;43(1):40–5.

Dental and Dentoalveolar Injuries in the Pediatric Patient

Harlyn K. Susarla, DMD, MPH*, Barbara Sheller, DDS, MSD

KEYWORDS

- Tooth fracture • Alveolar fracture • Tooth avulsion • Tooth luxation • Tooth displacement
- Dental injury

KEY POINTS

- Growth and development of the dentition and dental arches is critical to achieving optimal masticatory function and facial proportions.
- Injuries to the developing dentition merit prompt attention to determine the best management, based on the type of tooth injured (primary or permanent), dental age and development, chronologic age, and developmental age.
- Injuries to the primary teeth are typically managed by observation.
- Injuries to the permanent teeth may require more extensive interventions, based on time elapsed between injury and evaluation, type and extent of injury, and root maturity; all factors should be considered in the context of the patient's ability to cooperate for dental treatment.

INTRODUCTION

Traumatic dental and dentoalveolar injuries occur frequently in children and young adults. Although the oral cavity only represents 1% of the total body, injuries involving the oral cavity comprise 5% of all traumatic injuries.[1] The oral cavity is the second most common area of injury in children 0 to 6 years of age.[2] Approximately one-third of all adults have experienced permanent tooth trauma, most of which occurs by 19 years of age.[3] The most commonly injured teeth are maxillary incisors, which encompass 84% of primary tooth and 87% of permanent tooth injury.[4] Proper management of dental and dentoalveolar injuries is imperative to ensure the most favorable long-term outcome (**Fig. 1**). The information in this review uses the evidence-based guidelines set forth by the International Association of Dental Traumatology. The International Association of Dental Traumatology has a free app, "ToothSOS," which presents information to the public and to professionals about what to do after a dental injury.

A thorough history must be completed for any traumatic dental injury (TDI), including a basic assessment of airway, breathing, circulation, disability, and exposure, in accordance with Advanced Trauma Life Support parameters. Components include the time and place of injury, method of injury, potential for contamination of the injured structures, whether the injury was witnessed, and immediate interim management of the injury. Keep in mind that a young child is often unable to give a reliable history of the trauma event. As the clinician moves from the history to clinical evaluation, it is important to consider if the clinical findings are consistent with the history. If there is a concern for intentional injury or abuse, local protocols should immediately be followed.[3]

Critical items to address in the clinical evaluation are: identification of injured structures, type of management indicated, patient's ability to cooperate for the dental treatment, and recognition if a delay of hours or days before dental treatment will compromise the outcome. Comprehensive extraoral and intraoral examinations should

Department of Dentistry, Seattle Children's Hospital, 4800 Sand Point Way NE, Seattle, WA 98105, USA
* Corresponding author.
E-mail address: HARLYN.SUSARLA@SEATTLECHILDRENS.ORG

Oral Maxillofacial Surg Clin N Am 35 (2023) 543–554
https://doi.org/10.1016/j.coms.2023.06.002
1042-3699/23/© 2023 Elsevier Inc. All rights reserved.

oralmaxsurgery.theclinics.com

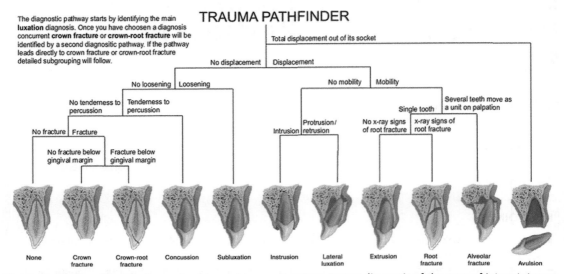

The diagnostic pathway starts by identifying the main **luxation** diagnosis. Once you have choosen a diagnosis concurrent **crown fracture** or **crown-root fracture** will be identified by a second diagnositic pathway. If the pathway leads directly to crown fracture or crown-root fracture detailed subgrouping will follow.

TRAUMA PATHFINDER

Fig. 1. Guide to assist with diagnosis of type of traumatic injury. Proper diagnosis of the type of injury is imperative to assist with appropriate management. (*From* Andreasen JO, Lauridsen E, Gerds TA, Ahrensburg SS. Dental Trauma Guide: a source of evidence-based treatment guidelines for dental trauma. Dent Traumatol. 2012;28(2):142-147.)

identify all hard and soft tissue injuries, including head injuries, fractures of the facial skeleton and/or alveolar processes, fractures or absence of teeth, alterations in occlusion, and any soft tissue lesions. Examination of the soft tissue should include an assessment for any embedded tooth fragments or other debris.[5]

Extraoral and intraoral photographs are recommended during the initial examination to establish a baseline.[6] Radiographic imaging should also be considered as appropriate for the type of injury, ability of the patient to cooperate for imaging, and radiographic resources available. Pulp sensibility tests are not recommended in primary teeth because they are not typically diagnostic;[5] however, such tests should be considered in the permanent dentition. Tooth position, displacement, mobility, integrity of crown, color, and tenderness to palpation and/or percussion should also be recorded.[5]

It is difficult to meet a patient for the first time when they have suffered a dental injury. It is important to add kindness and compassion to the provision of evidence-based treatment of TDI. Research into the cause of child dental fears has found that objective dental experiences play a minor role in fear acquisition, whereas subjective dental experiences seem to play the more decisive role.[6]

SPECIAL CONSIDERATIONS FOR PRIMARY TEETH

As children become more mobile, TDIs most commonly result from accidental falls, impacts,

and recreational activities.[7,8] These injuries occur most often between the ages of 2 and 6 years. Oftentimes, a TDI may result in a child's first dental visit and addressing potential anxiety of children and families is important. It may be helpful to examine uncooperative or precooperative children in a knee-to-knee position (**Fig. 2**).[9] These children should also be connected with a pediatric-oriented care team that offers the option of sedation or other behavior management techniques, additional treatment services if needed, and long-term follow-up.[5]

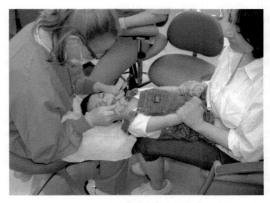

Fig. 2. Demonstration of the knee-to-knee position. The child is sitting in the parent's lap with their legs wrapped around the parent's waist. The child's head is supported in the practitioner's lap, while the parent holds the child's hand. The practitioner uses a toothbrush to help open the child's mouth when examining.

The buds of developing permanent teeth develop in close proximity to the apex of primary tooth. Trauma to a primary tooth may result in malformed, discolored, delayed, or impacted permanent successor teeth (**Fig. 3**).[10,11] Although the most common TDIs in the primary dentition are luxation injuries, intrusion and avulsion injuries of the primary dentition are most associated with development differences in permanent teeth.[3] The most serious complications occur when the child is younger than 2 years at the time of injury and with intrusion injuries.[12]

Unless there is an aspiration or ingestion risk, significant displacement of soft tissues (**Fig. 4**), a fractured tooth with a sharp edge that will cut the tongue or lip, or an occlusal interference where the teeth do not fit together, observation is typically the most appropriate choice during an emergency situation involving primary teeth.[13] For all primary TDI, parents/guardians should be instructed to: minimize further trauma to the area while supporting a return to normal function, provide a soft diet, and assist the child in cleaning the traumatized area with a soft toothbrush or a 0.1% to 0.2% alcohol-free chlorhexidine mouth rinse on a cotton swab two times a day for 1 week to minimize plaque accumulation and help facilitate healing.[5]

SPECIAL CONSIDERATIONS FOR PERMANENT TEETH

The most common TDIs in the permanent dentition are crown fractures (**Fig. 5**; see **Fig. 10**).[3] Preservation of pulp vitality in fractured immature permanent teeth allows root development to continue, improving chances of its long-term survival.[3] Losing a permanent tooth at any age is impactful, but losing a permanent tooth at a young age creates an additional burden when alveolar growth is affected and a malocclusion is created in an esthetic zone. As such, every attempt should be made to save the tooth.

Of all TDIs, avulsion of a permanent tooth is the most devastating. Prognosis is time-dependent; viability of the periodontal ligament (PDL) cells on the surface of the avulsed tooth root and maturity of the root determine tooth survival.[14] Patients and parents/guardians should be advised to minimize additional trauma to the area while supporting a return to normal function. Optimal home care decreases the bioburden and promotes favorable healing; the patient should be meticulous with oral hygiene and rinse with a 0.1% to 0.2% alcohol-free chlorhexidine solution or apply the solution on a cotton swab two times a day for 1 week to minimize plaque accumulation and help facilitate healing.[15]

FRACTURES OF THE TEETH

Fractures of the teeth include crown fractures, crown-root fractures, and root fractures. Determining the type and extent of a fracture through clinical and radiographic examination can help guide emergent and future treatment options.

Crown Fractures

Fractures involving the crown encompass 26.2% to 44.1% of all dental injuries.[16] Crown fractures are categorized either as uncomplicated or complicated. Uncomplicated crown fractures are enamel fractures or enamel-dentin fractures with no exposure of the pulp; complicated crown fractures involve enamel and dentin with exposure of the dental pulp (**Fig. 6**; see **Fig. 10**).[17]

Crown fractures do not usually present with discomfort to palpation or percussion.[18] In the case of tenderness, crown fractures should be assessed for luxation or root fracture injuries.[19] For any fracture involving the crown, one must evaluate for loose or missing tooth fragments.

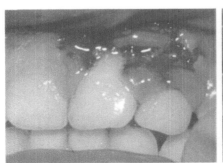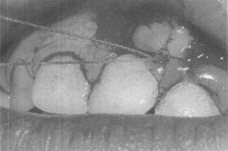

Fig. 3. Significant displacement of the soft tissue because of degloving of the gingiva apical to the primary central incisor. Such an injury may benefit from suture placement to assist in the reattachment of the gingiva while healing, and to protect the root of the primary incisor.

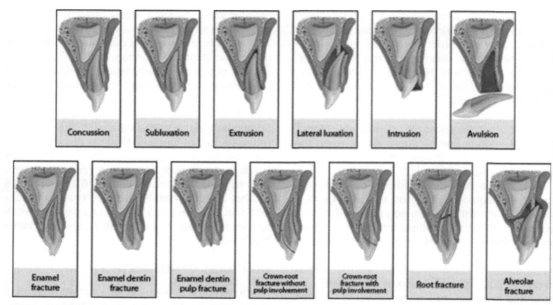

Fig. 4. Traumatic dental injuries in the primary dentition. The types of dental injuries sustained by primary teeth, and the proximity of the primary tooth to the developing permanent tooth bud is depicted here. Primary tooth trauma can result in developmental anomalies to the permanent tooth. The dental age of the child, and the type of trauma, are the two major factors that determine the effects on the permanent successor. (*From* Andreasen JO, Lauridsen E, Gerds TA, Ahrensburg SS. Dental Trauma Guide: a source of evidence-based treatment guidelines for dental trauma. Dent Traumatol. 2012;28(2):142-147.)

For missing tooth fragments in the setting of soft tissue injuries, radiographs should be taken to search for the fragments or any other foreign materials (including of the lip).[17] The exposed pulp in complicated crown fractures are sensitive to stimuli, such as cold air.

In primary teeth, a baseline radiograph is optional if the pulp is not exposed. If only the

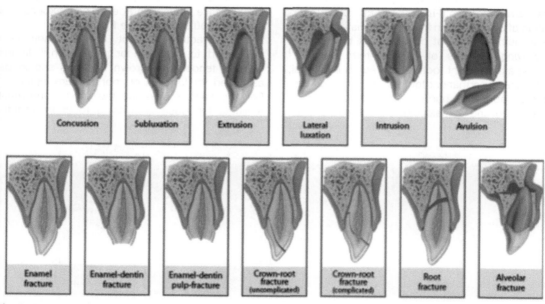

Fig. 5. Traumatic dental injuries of the permanent tooth. The types of injuries sustained by permanent teeth are depicted here. (*From* Andreasen JO, Lauridsen E, Gerds TA, Ahrensburg SS. Dental Trauma Guide: a source of evidence-based treatment guidelines for dental trauma. Dent Traumatol. 2012;28(2):142-147.)

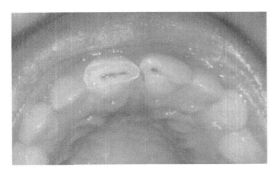

Fig. 6. Complicated crown fracture demonstrating pulp exposure of both maxillary central incisors.

enamel is fractured, any sharp edges may be smoothed. For enamel-dentin fractures, the exposed dentin should be covered with glass ionomer or composite. Missing tooth structure is restored at the initial visit or at a follow-up appointment, if needed.[5]

In permanent teeth, at least one periapical radiograph should be considered for any crown fractures to evaluate proximity to the nerve or to determine if any root fractures have occurred.[17] Additional radiographs should be considered in the setting of any other clinical signs or symptoms. In some cases, recovered tooth fragments of fractured permanent teeth may be bonded back to the tooth. Tooth fragments are rehydrated in water or saline for 20 minutes before reattachment. If tooth fragments cannot be found or saved, fractured edges are smoothed and restored with composite resin. For fractures within 0.5 mm of the pulp, a pink hue in the absence of frank bleeding is often visible in the fracture area. In these cases, calcium hydroxide or mineral trioxide aggregate may be placed on the dentin as a liner and covered with a glass ionomer or a similar material.

For complicated crown fractures in primary teeth, treatment depends on the child's ability to cooperate for dental treatment.[20] A radiograph should be taken. Ideally, the pulp should be preserved with a partial pulpotomy, using local anesthesia and nonsetting calcium hydroxide paste covered with a glass ionomer cement then restored with composite. Alternatively, no treatment may be the most appropriate option for a precooperative child or in a clinically unstable patient, with referral for immediate treatment to a child-oriented provider.[5]

In permanent teeth, complete root formation typically occurs approximately 4 years after eruption. Pulp vitality must be preserved in teeth with open apices or immature roots that have pulp exposures so that further root development can occur.[21,22] This is accomplished by using a partial pulpotomy or pulp capping. In mature teeth with full root formation, conservative therapy, such as a partial pulpotomy or placement of a nonsetting calcium hydroxide, mineral trioxide aggregate, or calcium silicate that does not stain, is also advised.[23] Root canal treatment is recommended for mature teeth with full root formation that require a post and core restoration.

Crown-Root Fractures

Crown-root fractures are fractures that often continue apical to the gingival margin. These fractures are of two types: uncomplicated or complicated crown-root fractures. Uncomplicated crown-root fractures are fractures of the enamel, dentin, and cementum without pulp exposure, whereas complicated crown-root fractures involve the enamel, dentin, cementum, and dental pulp.[17]

In primary teeth with either an uncomplicated or complicated crown-root fracture, a periapical or occlusal radiograph is recommended.[5] No treatment may be the appropriate option in an emergency, with referral for immediate treatment to a child-oriented provider. However, if treatment is considered at the time of the trauma, local anesthesia is needed. The loose fragment should be removed, and it should be determined if the crown is restorable. If it is restorable and there is no pulp exposure, glass ionomer is placed over exposed dentin. If a pulp exposure is apparent, a pulpotomy or root canal treatment is completed. If the tooth is nonrestorable, all readily accessible loose fragments should be extracted. To minimize damage to the developing permanent successor tooth bud, aggressive excavation of nonmobile pieces should be avoided.

In permanent teeth, one periapical radiograph and two additional radiographs at varying vertical and horizontal angulations should be taken. Cone beam computed tomography (CBCT) may also be used to obtain more precise information regarding the fractured area or amount of remaining tooth structure to better inform treatment options.[24] Any loose tooth fragments, which are usually present in crown-root fractures, should be temporarily stabilized, and missing fragments should be considered as in crown fractures.

For crown-root fractures, the overall treatment plan must take the patient's age and behavior into consideration. Options for future treatment may involve orthodontic or surgical extrusion, root canal treatment in the setting of an infected or necrotic pulp, root submergence, reimplantation, extraction, or autotransplantation.[17] Maintaining the tooth or a submerged root is favorable for alveolar growth and enhances the site for a future implant after skeletal maturity.

Root Fractures

Root fractures are horizontal and/or oblique fractures that involve the dentin, pulp, and cementum.[25] The coronal fragment is often mobile and displaced, and there may be occlusal interference. In primary teeth, the fracture is typically located either midroot or in the apical third of the root.[5] A periapical or occlusal radiograph is recommended to help localize the fracture. If there is no displacement of the coronal fragment, no treatment is necessary. If the fragment is displaced but not significantly mobile, the fragment should be left to spontaneously reposition itself, even in the presence of slight occlusal interference. If the coronal fragment is displaced, significantly mobile, or creating a significant occlusal interference, then the fragment may be extracted with local anesthesia, leaving the apical fragment to eventually resorb. Alternatively, the mobile coronal fragment may be repositioned and a passive and flexible splint placed for 4 weeks to stabilize it.[5]

Permanent teeth with root fractures may display percussion sensitivity and bleed from the gingival sulcus.[23] One periapical radiograph and two additional radiographs at varying vertical and horizontal angulations may help visualize the fracture. Sometimes, additional imaging, such as CBCT, may be needed to identify a root fracture that is not apparent on plain film, such as if the tooth has a nondisplaced vertical fracture.[23]

In root fractures, displaced coronal fragments should be promptly repositioned, and accurate repositioning should be confirmed with a radiograph. A passive and flexible splint should be placed for 4 weeks to stabilize the mobile coronal segment.[19] Stabilization for up to 4 months may be necessary for more cervically located fractures. Coronal segments should not be removed, because cervical fractures possess the capacity to heal. Endodontic treatment should not be started at the emergency visit. Both the fracture and condition of the pulp should be monitored for at least 1 year. Additional procedures may be needed in the future, depending on the maturity of the tooth and pulp status, including orthodontic or surgical extrusion of the apical segment, crown lengthening, root canal treatment in the setting of an infected or necrotic pulp, root submergence, or extraction.

Alveolar Process Fractures

Alveolar fractures, which extend from the buccal to the palatal bone in the maxilla, and the buccal to the lingual bony surface in the mandible, often present with mobility and displacement of a segment of teeth that move together.[17] An alveolar fracture may extend into the basal bone of the maxilla or mandible. Occlusal interferences may occur because of the positioning of the fractured segment. Displaced segments are repositioned and stabilized using the teeth as anchorage.

In primary teeth, a periapical or occlusal radiograph is recommended in addition to a lateral radiograph, which may provide information regarding any labial displacement of the segment.[5] Further imaging may also be necessary if it will impact the treatment plan. Using local anesthesia, the displaced alveolar segment should be repositioned and a passive and flexible splint should be placed for 4 weeks to stabilize as the bone heals.

In the permanent dentition, teeth within the fractured segment do not always react when the pulp is tested.[17] One periapical radiograph and two additional radiographs, at varying vertical and horizontal angulations, which sometimes includes an occlusal radiograph, may help visualize the fracture. A panoramic radiograph and/or CBCT can also be exposed if intraoral radiographs do not provide enough information to determine treatment.[23] After repositioning the fractured segment, a passive flexible splint should be placed for 4 weeks to stabilize (**Fig. 7**). Any apparent gingival lacerations may be sutured. It is not recommended to start root canal treatment at the emergency visit, and pulpal status should be monitored to determine if or when endodontic treatment may be needed.

DISPLACEMENT INJURIES
Concussion Injuries

Concussion injuries are where a tooth has undergone trauma (often being hit or bumped), and is sensitive to percussion and palpation.[17] However, no additional mobility or other abnormal clinical signs, and no radiographic injuries are present. In primary teeth, no treatment aside from observation is recommended, and no radiograph is advised unless an unfavorable outcome is suspected during follow-up. For permanent teeth, one periapical radiograph is recommended to confirm the diagnosis, but no treatment is needed. It is recommended to monitor the pulp condition in permanent teeth for at least 1 year, if not longer.

Subluxation Injuries

In subluxation injuries, a tooth that has undergone trauma is not displaced from its socket, but displays abnormal loosening and mobility.[14] These injuries present with a tooth that is sensitive to percussion and palpation, and sometimes demonstrate bleeding from the gingival sulcus.

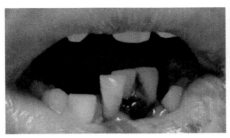 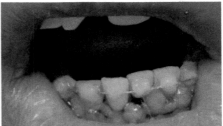

Fig. 7. Alveolar process fracture. Displacement of a segment of the mandibular incisors is seen in a 15-year-old boy after sustaining a blow to the face, and the subsequent stabilization of the mobile segment with the use of a passive and flexible splint.

In primary teeth, a periapical or occlusal radiograph is recommended, and demonstrates a normal or slightly widened PDL space. The treatment recommended is clinical monitoring via examination with radiographs taken at prescribed intervals.[5]

In permanent teeth, because transient pulp injury may be present, the tooth may initially be unresponsive to pulpal testing. One standard view periapical radiograph, supplemented by two additional radiographs at varying vertical and horizontal angulations, which sometimes include an occlusal radiograph, are recommended. Radiographic findings are often unremarkable. Typically, no treatment is necessary. If the subluxated tooth is excessively mobile, or exhibits tenderness when biting, a flexible passive splint may be placed for up to 2 weeks.[17] As in concussion injuries, it is recommended to monitor the pulp condition for at least a year, if not longer.

Extrusion/Extrusive Luxation Injuries

In extrusion injuries, the tooth has been axially displaced out of its socket (**Fig. 8**). Clinically, the tooth appears elongated and mobile.[17] Permanent teeth with extrusion injuries do not respond to pulpal testing. In radiographs, the extruded tooth appears elongated, not seated in the tooth socket, and the PDL space is increased in the apical direction for primary and permanent teeth, and also in the lateral direction for permanent teeth.

A periapical or occlusal radiograph is recommended for extruded primary teeth. Follow-up radiographs are only recommended in instances of pathosis.[5] Treatment is dependent on the amount of mobility, displacement, occlusal interference, root formation, and the child's ability to accept dental treatment. If no occlusal interference is present, the tooth should be given time to spontaneously reposition. In the case of excessive mobility of where the tooth is extruded more than 3 mm, extraction with local anesthesia under the guidance of a child-centered team with expertise in managing such injuries is recommended, because extractions in some patients have been associated with dental anxiety.[6]

For permanent teeth with extrusion injuries, one periapical radiograph and two additional radiographs, at varying vertical and horizontal angulations, which sometimes includes an occlusal radiograph, are recommended. After administering local anesthesia, the tooth should be repositioned gently into the socket, then stabilized with a flexible, passive splint for 2 weeks. If there is any fracture present of the marginal bone, the tooth should be splinted for 4 additional weeks. Vitality testing should be used to monitor the pulpal status. If necrosis or infection occur, appropriate endodontic treatment based on the root development of the tooth should be completed.

Lateral Luxation Injuries

In lateral luxation injuries, the tooth is displaced from its socket in a lateral direction, and is typically still partially attached to a segment of fractured alveolar bone.[17] The tooth is often immobile in lateral luxation injuries because of the bone fracture holding the apex in place. An occlusal interference may be present. A widened PDL space is apparent on either an occlusal radiograph or in periapical radiographs taken at different horizontal angles.

One periapical or occlusal radiograph is recommended for laterally luxated primary teeth. For primary teeth with minimal to no occlusal interference, the tooth should be given time to spontaneously reposition, which usually happens within 6 months. Teeth with severe displacement should be gently repositioned and stabilized with a flexible splint for 4 weeks. Extraction is appropriate when a laterally luxated tooth has significant mobility with risk of aspiration or ingestion.

Permanent teeth with lateral luxation injuries produce a high metallic tone on percussion, and

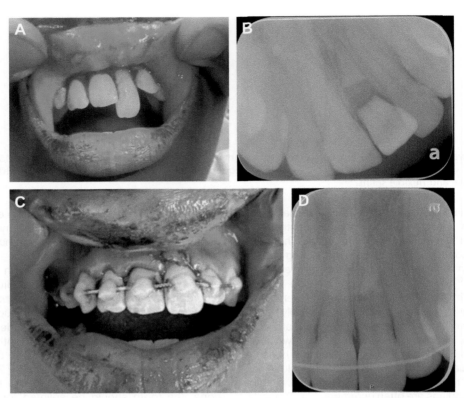

Fig. 8. (*A*) 16-year-old patient presenting with apparent extrusion and considerable mobility of the right lateral and bilateral central incisors, and subluxation of the left maxillary lateral incisor following assault. (*B*) Radiographically, the left maxillary central incisor has an associated mid-cervical horizontal root fracture with significant extrusion of the coronal fragment. (*C*) Following manual repositioning and non-rigid splint application there is improved arch alignment, though the left maxillary central incisor has a poor long-term prognosis given the horizontal root fracture and extent extrusion of the coronal fragment. (*D*) Radiographically, the extruded teeth have been repositioned, and the root fracture of the left maxillary incisor is reduced, as demonstrated by the discontinuity between its apical and cervical root fragments. The splint was maintained for 4 weeks, and endodontic follow-up was recommended within 2 weeks of injury.

typically is unresponsive to pulpal testing.[26] One periapical radiograph and two additional radiographs, at varying vertical and horizontal angulations, which sometimes includes an occlusal radiograph, are recommended. After administering local anesthesia, release the tooth from its fixed position and reposition it back into its socket. This is done by feeling the gingiva until the root apex is located, and using one digit to push in a downward direction over the apex, and another digit to guide the tooth into its socket. Stabilize the tooth with a passive flexible splint for at least 4 weeks. If a there is an associated fracture of the alveolar bone, extending the time of splinting may be warranted. Vitality testing should be used to monitor the pulpal status, beginning 2 weeks after the injury occurs. In teeth with incomplete root formation, spontaneous revascularization is possible; endodontic treatment should commence if necrosis or signs of infection-related external resorption occur. Pulp necrosis is

expected to occur in teeth with complete root formation. For mature teeth, staged root canal therapy should commence with the use of either a corticosteroid-antibiotic or with calcium hydroxide in the canal to decrease the occurrence of infection-related external resorption.

Intrusive Luxation

In intrusive luxation, the tooth is displaced apically into the alveolus, and is immobile.[27]

In primary teeth, the intruded tooth sometimes almost or completely disappears into the socket, and can damage the permanent tooth bud.[5] Although the tooth may not be visible, it can generally be palpated labially. One periapical or occlusal radiograph is recommended. If the apex has moved toward or through the buccal plate, it is visualized on radiograph and the tooth appears foreshortened compared with the contralateral tooth. If the apex has moved toward the permanent tooth bud, the tip cannot be seen on the image, and the tooth looks elongated.[28] The tooth should be given time to spontaneously re-erupt, regardless of position. This typically occurs within 6 months but can take up to 1 year.[29]

For intruded permanent teeth, a high metallic tone is heard on percussion, and the tooth typically is unresponsive to pulpal testing.[26,30] Radiographically, the PDL space may not be visualized, and the cementoenamel junction is positioned more apically than in adjacent teeth. One periapical radiograph and two additional radiographs, at varying vertical and horizontal angulations, which sometimes includes an occlusal radiograph, are recommended. Teeth with incomplete root formation should be given the chance to spontaneously re-erupt without outside intervention.[31] If there is no evidence of re-eruption within 4 weeks, orthodontic repositioning should be started. Spontaneous revascularization and pulpal healing of intruded immature teeth is possible, although endodontic treatment should commence if necrosis or signs of infection-related external resorption occur.

Management of intruded teeth with mature apices is determined by the degree of intrusion. Re-eruption without intervention should be planned when intrusion is less than 3 mm. If no re-eruption occurs within 8 weeks intervention should be started before progression of ankylosis. The tooth should be either surgically repositioned and stabilized with a passive flexible splint for 4 weeks, or it should be orthodontically repositioned. Teeth intruded 3 to 7 mm, should be surgically repositioned, although orthodontic repositioning is also acceptable as a secondary option. Teeth intruded more than 7 mm should be surgically repositioned.[17] Necrosis is expected to occur in intruded teeth with complete root formation. Root canal therapy should commence within 2 weeks with the use of either a corticosteroid-antibiotic or with calcium hydroxide in the canal to decrease the occurrence of infection-related external resorption.

Tooth Avulsions

In an avulsion, the tooth is entirely out of the socket (**Figs. 9** and **10**). The location of the missing tooth should be determined. The impact of the avulsion injury may displace the tooth extraorally, into the oral soft tissues or nose, into the esophagus, or into the respiratory tract.[15] When an avulsed tooth cannot be located, the patient should be evaluated in an emergency room, particularly in the instance of potential respiratory sequelae.

Avulsed primary teeth should not be reimplanted to minimize damage to the developing permanent successor tooth.[5]

In permanent teeth, 0.5% to 16% of all TDI consist of avulsion injuries.[32] One of the most serious and potentially devastating dental injuries that occurs, prognosis following avulsion is time-dependent. Reimplantation of the avulsed tooth is the preferred treatment in nearly all situations. Among the contraindications to reimplantation are: avulsed tooth is defective/carious, periodontal disease is present, patient is immunosuppressed, and/or the patient's behavior does not allow for reimplantation.[15]

To preserve vitality of PDL cells on the root surface, the tooth should be handled only by the crown (white portion of the tooth that resembles the tooth clinically) and the tooth should be immediately reimplanted. If the tooth is visibly contaminated, it may be gently rinsed in milk, saline, or the patient's saliva before being reimplanted. The patient should bite on gauze or a napkin after reimplantation and continue biting while being transported to a dentist for evaluation and splinting.[33]

If immediate reimplantation is not feasible, the tooth should be placed in the following storage media in order of preference: cold milk, Hanks balanced salt solution, saliva, or saline.[34] If none of these are available, the tooth should be placed in water rather than allowed to become dry. However, water is an inferior option because it causes lysis of the PDL cells.[35] The patient and tooth should then be brought to a dental professional immediately.

The treatment of avulsion injuries depends on root maturity, and the state of the PDL cells. Root maturity is determined by whether the root has an open or closed apex.[36]

The long-term prognosis of the tooth is determined by the vitality of the PDL cells, which are affected by the extraoral dry time of the tooth and the storage medium in which the tooth was transported. Because most PDL cells typically die after 30 minutes of extraoral dry time, minimizing dry time is extremely important.[15] If the tooth is replanted within 15 minutes at the location of the trauma, the PDL cells are likely viable. If the extraoral dry time is less than 60 minutes and the tooth has been placed in a storage medium, some PDL cells may be viable, although compromised. The PDL cells for teeth not placed in a storage medium that have an extraoral dry time that is greater than 60 minutes are likely not viable.

If an avulsed permanent tooth has been replanted at the location of the trauma or before seeing a specialist, the injured area should first

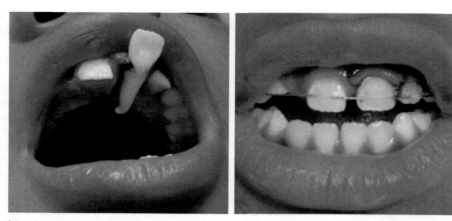

Fig. 9. Avulsion in an 8 year old. Tooth #9 is completely avulsed from its socket, but still attached to the gingiva. Tooth was reimplanted with a flexible splint, which was extended from primary canine to primary canine.

be cleaned with water, saline, or chlorhexidine. The position of the tooth should be confirmed through clinical and radiographic examination. The tooth should be left in place or slightly repositioned with light digital pressure, if needed. Teeth that are rotated or placed into the wrong socket may be repositioned into their correct location for up to 48 hours after the trauma occurred. The tooth should then be stabilized with a passive, flexible splint for at least 2 weeks (see **Fig. 9**). A more rigid splint may be used for up to 4 weeks if there is an associated alveolar fracture.[15,37]

If the extraoral dry time of an avulsed tooth is less than 60 minutes and the tooth has been placed in a storage medium, the tooth should be examined, and debris should be removed gently either in the storage medium or by rinsing with

sterile saline.[15] Local anesthesia, preferably without a vasoconstrictor, should be used, and the socket should then be irrigated with sterile saline. Remove any coagulum present in the socket, and reposition any fractured segments of the socket wall before tooth replantation. The tooth should then be stabilized with a passive flexible splint for at least 2 weeks. Replant the tooth slowly using light digital pressure, and confirm correct position clinically and radiographically. A more rigid splint may be used for up to 4 weeks if there is an associated alveolar fracture.

If extraoral dry time is greater than 60 minutes, the same guidelines should be followed as for avulsed teeth with less than 60 minute dry time.[15] However, the patient and family should be informed that these teeth have a poor long-

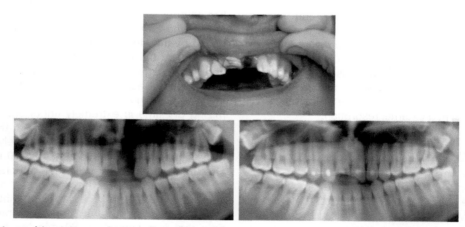

Fig. 10. An avulsion injury and a complicated crown fracture are present in this 17 year old after an injury when swimming. The radiograph on the left reveals a complete avulsion of the right maxillary central incisor, and a complicated crown fracture of the left central incisor. The avulsed tooth was subsequently reimplanted, and a flexible splint was placed, with instructions for the patient to subsequently follow-up with their dentist for further treatment and evaluation.

term prognosis because of the delay in replantation, because the PDL will become necrotic. It is expected that these teeth will have ankylosis-related root resorption. The reason for replantation of teeth with a poor long-term prognosis is to temporarily reestablish form and function and maintain the alveolar bone in this area for future treatment options.

Systemic antibiotics, such as amoxicillin or penicillin, are recommend after an avulsion of a permanent tooth to decrease the risk of reactions from infection and to decrease the risk of inflammatory root resorption.[38] Topical antibiotics on the root surface are no longer recommended. Tetanus status should also be checked because of the potential for contamination at the location of the trauma.[39]

Patients with replanted teeth should be instructed to avoid contact sports, follow a soft food diet for 2 weeks, brush with a soft toothbrush, and use a 0.12% chlorhexidine mouth rinse two times a day for 2 weeks.[15]

For avulsed teeth with open apices and a brief extraoral time, there is a chance that pulpal revascularization may occur.[36] As such, root canal therapy should not commence unless there is clinical or radiographic evidence of pulpal necrosis. For teeth with closed apices, root canal therapy should commence within 2 weeks of the injury.

SUMMARY

Although TDI are common and frequently present as isolated injuries, they can have substantial long-term consequences. Careful assessment of the patient, including a full evaluation of the facial skeleton and sensorium, is paramount to appropriate diagnosis and tailored management, based on patient age and dental development. TDIs are classified as injuries to the tooth proper (crown fractures, crown-root fractures, and root fractures), injuries altering the position of the tooth (intrusion, extrusion, and luxation injuries), and injuries to the alveolar housing (alveolar fractures). Management of these injuries is predicated on an understanding of the normal sequence of dental development and facial growth. Successful treatment results not only from timely assessment and initial management, but also longitudinal follow-up.

CLINICS CARE POINTS

- Most primary tooth injuries are treated conservatively with observation.

- Injuries to permanent teeth may require specific treatments to address injuries to the tooth structure or position.
- Following initial treatment, long-term follow-up is necessary to determine the optimal treatment plan to achieve a functional occlusion as the dentoalveolar structures and facial skeleton continue to grow.

REFERENCES

1. Andersson L. Epidemiology of traumatic dental injuries. Pediatr Dent 2013;35(2):102–5.
2. Petersson EE, Andersson L, Sorensen S. Traumatic oral vs non-oral injuries. Swed Dent J 1997;21:55–68.
3. Levin L, Day PF, Hicks L, et al. International Association of Dental Traumatology guidelines for the management of traumatic dental injuries: general introduction. Dent Traumatol 2020;36(4):309–13.
4. Lombardi SM, Sheller B, Williams BJ. Diagnosis and treatme tof dental trauma in a children's hospital. Pediatr Dent 1998;20:2 112–120.
5. Day PF, Flores MT, O'Connell AC, et al. International Association of Dental Traumatology guidelines for the management of traumatic dental injuries: 3. Injuries in the primary dentition. Dent Traumatol 2020;36(4):343–59.
6. Ten Berge M, Veerkamp JSJ, Hoogstraten J. The etiology of childhood dental fear; the role of dental and conditioning experiences. J. Anxiety Disord 2002; 16:321–9.
7. Andersson L, Petti S, Day P, et al. Classification, epidemiology and etiology. In: Andreasen JO, Andreasen FM, Andersson L, editors. Textbook and color atlas of traumatic injuries to the teeth. 5th edition. Copenhagen: Wiley Blackwell; 2019. p. 252–94.
8. Andreasen JOAF, Bakland LK, Flores MT. Traumatic dental injuries, a manual. 3rd edition. Chichester, UK: Wiley-Blackwell; 2011.
9. Myers GL. Evaluation and diagnosis of the traumatized dentition. Dent Traumatol 2019;35(6):302–8.
10. Flores MT, Onetto JE. How does orofacial trauma in children affect the developing dentition? Long-term treatment and associated complications. Dent Traumatol 2019;35:312–23.
11. Lenzi MM, Alexandria AK, Ferreira DM, et al. Does trauma in the primary dentition cause sequelae in permanent successors? A systematic review. Dent Traumatol 2015;31:79–88.
12. von Arx T. Developmental disturbances of permanent teeth following trauma to the primary dentition. Aust Dent J 1993;38(1):1–10.
13. Flores MT, Holan G, Andreasen JO, et al. Injuries to the primary dentition. In: Andreasen JO, Andreasen FM, Andersson L, editors. Textbook and color atlas of

traumatic injuries to the teeth. 5th edition. Copenhagen, Denmark: Wiley Blackwell; 2019. p. 556–88.

14. Andreasen JO. Effect of extra-alveolar period and storage media upon periodontal and pulpal healing after replantation of mature permanent incisors in monkeys. Int J Oral Surg 1981;10:43–53.

15. Fouad AF, Abbott PV, Tsilingaridis G, et al. International Association of Dental Traumatology guidelines for the management of traumatic dental injuries: 2. Avulsion of permanent teeth. Dent Traumatol 2020;36(4):331–42.

16. Marinčák D, Doležel V, Přibyl M, et al. Conservative treatment of complicated crown fracture and crown-root fracture of young permanent incisor: a case report with 24-month follow-up. Children 2021;8(9):725.

17. Bourguignon C, Cohenca N, Lauridsen E, et al. International Association of Dental Traumatology guidelines for the management of traumatic dental injuries: 1. Fractures and luxations. Dent Traumatol 2020;36(4):314–30.

18. Robertson A. A retrospective evaluation of patients with uncomplicated crown fractures and luxation injuries. Endod Dent Traumatol 1998;14(6):245–56.

19. Molina JR, Vann WF Jr, McIntyre JD, et al. Root fractures in children and adolescents: diagnostic considerations. Dent Traumatol 2008;24:503–9.

20. American Academy of Pediatric Dentistry. Behaviour guidance for the pediatric dental patient. Pediatr Dent 2015;40:254–67.

21. Bimstein E, Rotstein I. Cvek pulpotomy: revisited. Dent Traumatol 2016;32:438–42.

22. Andreasen JO, Bakland LK, Andreasen FM. Traumatic intrusion of permanent teeth. Part 2. A clinical study of the effect of preinjury and injury factors, such as sex, age, stage of root development, tooth location, and extent of injury including number of intruded teeth on 140 intruded permanent teeth. Dent Traumatol 2006;22(2):90–8.

23. Cvek M. Prognosis of luxated non-vital maxillary incisors treated with calcium hydroxide and filled with gutta percha. Endod Dent Traumatol 1992;8:45–55.

24. Cohenca N, Silberman A. Contemporary imaging for the diagnosis and treatment of traumatic dental injuries: a review. Dent Traumatol 2017;33:321–8.

25. Abbott PV. Diagnosis and management of transverse root fractures. Dent Traumatol 2019;35(6):333–47.

26. Lauridsen E, Hermann NV, Gerds TA, et al. Combination injuries 3. The risk of pulp necrosis in permanent teeth with extrusion or lateral luxation and concomitant crown fractures without pulp exposure. Dent Traumatol 2012;28:379–85.

27. Andreasen JO, Bakland LK, Andreasen FM. Traumatic intrusion of permanent teeth. Part 3. A clinical study of the effect of treatment variables such as treatment delay, method of repositioning, type of splint, length of splinting and antibiotics on 140 teeth. Dental Traumatol 2006;22:99–111.

28. Holan G, Ram D. Sequelae and prognosis of intruded primary incisors: a retrospective study. Pediatr Dent 1999;21(4):242–7.

29. Lauridsen E, Blanche P, Yousaf N, et al. The risk of healing complications in primary teeth with intrusive luxation: a retrospective cohort study. Dent Traumatol 2017;33:329–36.

30. Andreasen JO, Bakland LK, Matras RC, et al. Traumatic intrusion of permanent teeth. Part 1. An epidemiological study of 216 intruded permanent teeth. Dent Traumatol 2006;22(2):83–9.

31. Hurley E, Stewart C, Gallagher C, et al. Decisions on repositioning of intruded permanent incisors; a review and case presentation. Eur J Paediatr Dent 2018;19(2):101–4.

32. DiPaolo M, Townsend J, Peng J, et al. Characteristics, treatment outcomes and direct costs of tooth avulsion in children treated at a major hospital. Dent Traumatol 2023;39(3):240–7.

33. Flores MT, Andersson L, Andreasen JO, et al. Guidelines for the management of traumatic dental injuries. Ii. Avulsion of permanent teeth. Dent Traumatol 2007;23:130–6.

34. Adnan S, Lone MM, Khan FR, et al. Which is the most recommended medium for the storage and transport of avulsed teeth? A systematic review. Dent Traumatol 2018;34:59–70.

35. Is Khinda V, Kaur G, S Brar G, et al. Clinical and practical implications of storage media used for tooth avulsion. Int J Clin Pediatr Dent 2017;10(2):158–65.

36. Kahler B, Rossi-Fedele G, Chugal N, et al. An evidence-based review of the efficacy of treatment approaches for immature permanent teeth with pulp necrosis. J Endod 2017;43(7):1052–7.

37. Andreasen JO. Periodontal healing after replantation of traumatically avulsed human teeth: assessment by mobility testing and radiography. Acta Odontol Scand 1975;33:325–35.

38. Hammarstrom L, Blomlof L, Feiglin B, et al. Replantation of teeth and antibiotic treatment. Endod Dent Traumatol 1986;2:51–7.

39. Rhee P, Nunley MK, Demetriades D, et al. Tetanus and trauma: a review and recommendations. J Trauma 2005;58:1082–8.

Pediatric Mandible Fractures

Jeffrey Hajibandeh, DDS, MD*, Zachary S. Peacock, DMD, MD

KEYWORDS

- Pediatric mandible fracture • Jaw fracture • Pediatric injuries • Malocclusion • Growth disturbance

KEY POINTS

- Pediatric facial fractures are uncommon; the mandible is the most commonly fractured facial bone. Many pediatric mandible fractures can be managed nonsurgically or with closed techniques.
- Available data suggest similar outcomes between closed versus open treatment.
- Open treatment may be warranted in cases of severe displacement, multiple fractures, or inability to tolerate intermaxillary fixation.

BACKGROUND

Craniomaxillofacial surgeons managing pediatric mandible fractures should have a general understanding of growth and development of the pediatric facial skeleton, which also helps contextualize the statistics surrounding pediatric mandible fractures. Growth cessation of the mandible occurs later than all other facial bones (age 14–16 years in females; 18–20 years in males).[1,2] The condyle is believed to be a primary growth center of the mandible,[3] and the damage during periods of active growth may lead to significant growth disturbance.[2,4] Fortunately, many factors reduce the frequency of mandibular fractures in children as compared with adults. From infancy through the mixed dentition, the cranium is proportionally larger than the face providing relative protection against facial injuries. Bone in children has a lower elastic modulus than adults, decreasing the frequency of fractures. Tooth buds during the primary and mixed dentition comprise most of the volume of the developing mandible and are thought to be protective against fractures. Common fracture patterns in pediatric patients include incomplete or "green stick" injuries where cortical violation may be unilateral and incomplete. These biomechanical considerations may explain why facial fractures in children are often associated with other injuries, morbidity, and mortality.[5]

EPIDEMIOLOGY

Several institutional-based studies describe epidemiology and demographics surrounding mandible fractures. The most common mechanisms of injury are motor vehicle collisions[6] followed closely by assault/abuse, mechanical falls, and sports-related injuries.[6–8] As in adults, there is a strong male predilection and the average age is 9 to 12 years.[9,10] Dental crown fracture and tooth avulsion commonly occur with pediatric mandible fractures.[11] The most common pediatric mandibular fracture location overall in children is the mandibular condyle/subcondylar region[12–14] followed by the symphysis, but the predominance varies by age and mandibular development.[10] Children less than 8 years more commonly have condylar head fractures, but after this, the condylar neck enlarges and condylar neck fractures predominate.[14] Mandibular body and angle fractures become more common as the mandible completes development.[15]

Owusu and colleagues conducted a review of the Healthcare Cost and Utilization Project–Nationwide Emergency Department Sample, a comprehensive database available for emergency department encounters in the United States. Their study corroborated previous institutional and regional studies. They also reported a male predilection (4:1) and consistent age-related

Massachusetts General Hospital, Division of Oral & Maxillofacial Surgery, Warren 1201, 55 Fruit Street, Boston, MA 02127, USA
* Corresponding author.
E-mail address: jhajibandeh@partners.org

Oral Maxillofacial Surg Clin N Am 35 (2023) 555–562
https://doi.org/10.1016/j.coms.2023.05.001
1042-3699/23/

distribution and location of fracture (condyle fractures as the most common site of injury overall [14%]). Condylar fractures were most common less than 12 years old secondary to falls, whereas greater than 12, fractures of the angle of the mandible predominated. In addition, they found a relationship between anatomic site and gender; males were more likely to have angle fractures (15%), whereas females had more condylar fractures (20%).[12]

CLINICAL ASSESSMENT

Initial evaluation and management follows advanced traumatic life support protocols for identification and management of life-threatening injuries. Mandible fractures in children are commonly associated with intracranial and/or cervical spine injuries. In-line stabilization of the cervical spine should be maintained during evaluation and operative management if injuries are suspected or cannot be ruled out.[10,12] In children, standard history and physical examination can be limited by an inability to describe symptoms such as pain, vision changes, or malocclusion. Assessment should be done with the input of caregivers where appropriate. A thorough physical examination is warranted assessing for predictors of facial fractures. Soft tissue injuries including swelling, laceration, or ecchymoses may provide a gauge of injury severity.[16] Concomitant dentoalveolar injuries occur in nearly 25% of pediatric mandible fracture[17] with tooth avulsion representing the most common associated injury.[18] Any teeth unaccounted for require imaging to rule out aspiration. The clinician should determine the child's dentition pattern (primary, mixed, or adult), inspect for soft tissue injuries extra- and intraorally that can indicate adjacent fractures. Examination findings vary by fracture location but can include malocclusion, step-offs in the inferior border or dentition, mobility of fracture segments, trismus, deviation to the ipsilateral side on opening, and paresthesia of the lower lip and/or chin.

IMAGING

Imaging studies to assess fracture patterns may include two-dimensional (2D) plain film or 3D studies. Plain x-ray imaging (eg, panoramic radiograph or facial series) has several limitations in the pediatric population that may lead to a misdiagnosis: (1) presence of tooth buds, overlap of anatomic structures, and the developing ramus–condylar units may obscure visualization of fracture patterns and (2) limited patient compliance may introduce motion artifact preventing accurate diagnosis. Computed tomography (CT) imaging is widely accepted as the clinical gold standard for patients sustaining facial trauma for its 3D visualization of fracture patterns. In children, CT imaging more reliably detects fractures with greater sensitivity and specificity compared with panoramic imaging, especially for condylar fractures.[19] Given concerns about ionizing radiation in the growing patient, clinicians should adhere to ALARA (as low as reasonably achievable) principles.[20,21] MRI has been applied recently for children sustaining trauma.[22] MRI may provide suitable sensitivity and specificity for diagnosis of mandible fractures while eliminating radiation, but more studies are needed.[23] Limitations include a lack of 3D skeletal images and longer acquisition time which could result in motion artifact and/or necessitate sedation in young patients.

MANAGEMENT

The goal of treatment for mandibular fractures is to restore mandibular form and function and minimize growth disturbance. Factors to consider include patient age, fracture pattern, degree of displacement, risk for growth disturbance, and ability to comply with instructions.[24] Owing to these factors, pediatric facial fractures have increasingly been managed at tertiary medical centers.[5]

Nonsurgical or closed treatment of pediatric mandible fractures has long been an accepted treatment pattern where there is minimal change in occlusion or fractures are non-displaced.[25,26] Factors in favor of this treatment option include rapid healing, potential for occlusal correction with eruption of permanent teeth, growth compensation, and avoidance of the operative risks of open treatment.[27] In addition, sustaining a mandible fracture has not been correlated with need for future orthodontic treatment.[28] For non-displaced fractures, without malocclusion or limitation in opening can be managed by a limited diet (ie, blenderized), analgesics, and close observation.[29] Advancement to soft foods and early return of function is emphasized to prevent limited mouth opening or temporomandibular joint (TMJ) ankylosis. Gentle jaw-opening exercises are added shortly after diagnosis particularly with intracapsular condylar fractures. Children in the primary or mixed dentition with a minor malocclusion have the potential for dental compensation may also be managed with nonsurgical treatment.

Children with malocclusion or displacement of fractures usual require surgical intervention. Closed treatment (ie, maxillomandibular fixation [MMF]) can be instituted in mild/moderate displacement.[30] Severely displaced fractures or those that cannot be reduced using closed techniques require open treatment which can include reduction and internal fixation. Some cases may require a combination of open reduction internal fixation with closed treatment[31] such as a displaced body fracture and condylar fracture (**Fig. 1**).

Closed Versus Open Treatment Techniques

Closed treatment serves to immobilize or guide the mandible to the patients' premorbid occlusal relationship to help maintain bony anatomic reduction. Advantages include the decreased risk of iatrogenic injury associated with periosteal stripping for exposure,[32] damage to tooth buds or need for subsequent hardware removal. In the pediatric population, the state of the dentition (primary, adult, mixed) must be assessed as this will influence the choice of intermaxillary fixation. The traditional circumdental wiring using Eric arch bars may not be feasible in the primary or early mixed dentition where bulbous crowns with lower height of contour limit retention of wires and adaptability of an arch bar. Risdon cables (braided 26-gauge wires secured with circumdental wires) better adapt to primary teeth and allow wired MMF[33] (**Fig. 2**). Occasionally preexisting orthodontic appliances can be used for elastic or wire maxillomandibular guidance or fixation.[34] If circumdental wiring is not possible (eg, multiple missing teeth), circummandibular wiring can provide stability and reliable outcomes.[35] Occlusal and lingual splints can be used for additional stability when the dentition is limited. A lingual splint (either made preoperatively or intraoperatively using thermoplastic material) can help establish the width of the mandible with a symphysis fracture and can be used with closed and as an adjunct to open treatment[36] (**Fig. 3**).

Closed treatment duration should be shorter in children as compared with adults. For children in the primary or mixed dentition, rarely is more than 2 weeks of MMF necessary.[29] Gentle stretching exercises should be prescribed after MMF to regain motion particularly with fractures of the condyle with observation of the amount of opening over several months.

The use of progressively remodeled splints combined with fixed orthodontic appliances can lead to satisfactory TMJ function in patients with mixed dentition.[37] There are however age-determinant outcomes associated with closed treatment. The closed treatment of condylar fractures in older children (>12 years of age) has higher rates of posttreatment malocclusion, TMJ dysfunction, and mandibular deviation. In addition, they have more persistent radiographic changes of ramus–condylar morphology.[38]

Open treatment may be indicated when there is significant fracture displacement, bilateral injuries, or adolescents with condylar neck injuries.[29] When open treatment is used, plate and screw fixation should be placed along the inferior border of the mandible to avoid damage to unerupted teeth and dental follicles.[14] When tooth follicles occupy a large vertical proportion of the body space and fixation is needed, monocortical fixation with short screws should be used. Theoretically, fixation should not cross the midsagittal plane as it may restrict growth.[39] The position of the inferior alveolar nerve (IAN) also changes during development and should be accounted for when placing fixation. Initially, the IAN is positioned inferior-lingually and progressing superiorly toward the middle of the mandible.[29]

Open treatment of pediatric mandible fractures can be achieved with a variety of materials for rigid osteosynthesis. Most surgeons prefer the use of titanium as for familiarity given use in adults, biocompatibility, accessibility, and ease of

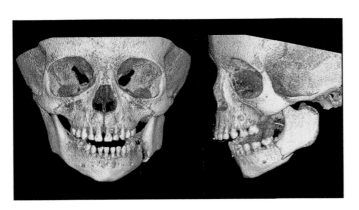

Fig. 1. Frontal and lateral oblique views of a 3 year old with a left mandibular body and subcondylar fracture. Note the primary dentition with bulbous crowns and generalized interdental spacing.

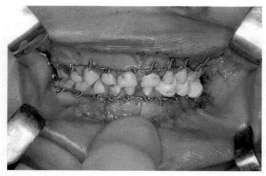

Fig. 2. Risdon cables composed of braided 26-gauge wires secured with circumdental wires used to facilitate intermaxillary fixation. Note the Blu-Mousse (Parkell, Inc, Edgewood, NY, USA) in the left occlusal surfaces used to open the bite posteriorly to try to reestablish the ramus–condylar height.

adaptation to the skeleton.[8] Titanium osteosynthesis is biomechanically superior to resorbable systems and less technique sensitive. Concerns of growth restriction or translocation of hardware medially and posteriorly with growth has led to planned removal or use of resorbable plating systems.

Resorbable osteosynthesis can be used for some mandible fractures. They offer the theoretical advantage of less growth disturbance and can avoid a second operation for removal.[40]

Resorbable plating systems are commonly made from polymers of polyglycolic and poly-L-lactic acid that require several months to dissolve. They may require pre-tapping after drilling screw holes. Fixation with resorbable plates should be applied in a load-sharing manner due to less fixation strength.[41] Some surgeons therefore combine a short period of MMF with the use of resorbable plating techniques.[31] Unlike titanium plates, resorbable plates have poor memory and therefore do not provide reliable contouring or overreduction.[29] Previous studies have demonstrated no significant difference in rates of infection between resorbable and titanium plates.[41,42]

Symphysis and body fractures
As tooth buds are protective, fractures due to direct trauma to the symphysis and body occur more commonly in older children. Most fractures are non-displaced and favorable.[43] Children sustaining an isolated and nonmobile fracture may be managed with observation and limited diet. Close monitoring is recommended to allow intervention with changes in the fracture or occlusion.[44]

With mobility or displacement, closed treatment or open reduction internal fixation (ORIF) should be used.[34] A single plate can be placed at the inferior border along with stabilization of the dentition using arch bars or Risdon cables (see **Fig. 3**). As above, width can be restored using a lingual splint

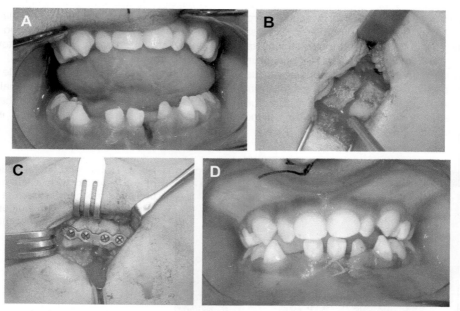

Fig. 3. Open reduction internal fixation of a 3 year old with a body fracture. (*A*) Clinical examination demonstrating a gingival laceration with diastasis, (*B*) transcervical exposure, (*C*) fixation using a single miniplate with four monocortical screws, and (*D*) closure of the intraoral laceration. (*Courtesy of* Srinivas M. Susarla, DMD, MD, MPH, [Seattle, WA].)

(Fig. 4); "Tension bands" should not be used due to developing teeth. The dental fixation can be removed 4 to 6 weeks after fixation and the plate if indicated removed after 4 to 6 months.

Angle fractures

As opposed to adults, mandibular angle fractures in children are uncommon (only 4% of mandibular fractures in children < 12 years old).[12] Nondisplaced and nonmobile fractures may be treated with observation or closed treatment. With displacement or mobility, no consensus for treatment exists. Closed treatment has been reported to be successful but other investigators advocate ORIF to counter biomechanical forces displacing angle fractures.[45,46]

A few small studies have looked at angle fractures in children. The largest series is 17 subjects over a 30-year period.[46] Of these, nine underwent ORIF with only four in the primary/mixed dentition. The use of a single miniplate had less complications including plate exposure or effect on developing molars as opposed to larger or multiple plates. Additional studies support the use of a single miniplate for angle fractures in children.[47]

Condylar fractures

The most common mandibular fracture in children occurs in the condyle. A fall on the chin can result in force superiorly resulting in fractures of the head or neck of the condyle. Depending on the orientation of the force, fractures can be unilateral or bilateral. The greatest risk for growth disturbance occurs in these injuries. Missed diagnoses or inappropriate treatment can result in undergrowth of one or both condyles resulting in asymmetry or retrognathia. Excessive immobilization can result in limited motion and ankylosis of the condyle to the skull base. Children less than 6 years of age sustaining intracapsular condylar injuries are at high risk for ankylosis particularly those less than 3 years.[48]

Children in the primary or mixed dentition sustaining condylar head fractures can generally be treated with a soft diet and regular follow-up. Jaw motion exercises can be started within a few days of the injury and range of motion should be assessed at each visit. Manual stretching with parents or the use of commercially available devices may be needed.

With the presence of a malocclusion, displacement, or dislocation, surgical treatment should be considered. Closed treatment using guiding elastics may achieve correction of occlusion and jaw deviation and generally allows remodeling of the adaptable pediatric condyle.[49] Residual malocclusions have the potential for correction with alveolar bone growth and eruption of the permanent dentition. Some surgeons advocate a short period of MMF, whereas others recommend guiding elastics only. Closed reduction with MMF should be limited to 1 to 3 weeks with recent studies recommending no more than 10 days to facilitate a return to function.[50,51] Tabrizi and colleagues[52] prospectively compared MMF with guiding elastics and found no difference in outcomes including jaw opening, deviation, or TMJ dysfunction. Guiding elastics were more tolerable and therefore recommended by the investigators.

Studies have assessed radiographic outcomes of nonsurgical or closed treatment of condylar fractures. Children under 12 years have the greatest potential to achieve remodeling of the condyle to a normal condyle/fossa relationship.[53,54] Remodeling typically occurs within 2 to 3 years of the injury.[53,55]

ORIF is rarely used for pediatric condylar fractures. Clear indications include perforation of the condyle through the glenoid fossa, external auditory canal, or with concomitant midface fractures requiring restoration of vertical height of the condyle ramus unit as reference.[56] Relative indications include inadequate outcomes with closed treatment, severely displaced fractures especially for children with adult dentition (>12 years of age) with less remodeling/adaptive capacity.[57,58]

Long-Term Outcomes

Growth disturbance and facial deformity are the most severe long-term complications that can occur with mandibular fractures in childhood. Condyle fractures are the most common injury that leads to facial asymmetry in children.[28] Lund performed the only long-term prospective study

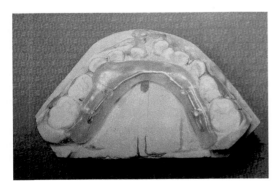

Fig. 4. Lingual splints fabricated for the purposes of closed treatment of a mandible fracture created from a study model. (*From* Susarla SM, Peacock ZS. Chapter 81: Pediatric Mandibular Fractures. In: Tiwana, PS, Kademani, D, eds. Atlas of Oral and Maxillofacial Surgery. 2nd ed. Elsevier; 2024:880–886.)

of children with condylar fractures.[59] In 27 children with unilateral condylar fractures, 78% exhibited compensatory growth (ie, greater growth of the fractured condyle compared with the uninjured side). In many cases (30%), the fractured side grew enough to overcome an existing asymmetry, but others (48%) did not "overgrow" enough to overcome an asymmetric condyle–ramus unit. In 22%, growth lagged the uninjured side and the asymmetry worsened over time. Younger patients experienced the most compensatory growth, whereas those near the end or after the pubertal growth spurt had less growth and more asymmetry. Frequently, growth disturbances may be managed by interceptive orthodontics or orthognathic surgery at the end of growth. Demianczuk and colleagues showed that children who sustained mandibular fractures before 4 years of age or after 12 years were unlikely to require orthognathic surgery. Children with fractures between 4 and 11 years (mixed dentition) frequently (17–22%) had orthognathic surgery.[28]

Ankylosis of the TMJ is a rare but devastating complication of mandibular fractures in children.[60] Condylar head (intracapsular) fractures with extended periods of immobilization are high risk, but any condylar fracture in children under age 3 years has risk of ankylosis.[61–63] TMJ ankylosis presents with profound limitations in motion and results in severely limited growth, asymmetry, or mandibular retrognathia. Diagnosis requires CT imaging, and management is beyond the scope of this article.

SUMMARY

Pediatric mandibular fractures are uncommon as compared with adults and require special considerations. Many injuries can be treated with nonsurgical or closed treatment; however, open treatment with fixation can be indicated. In children, long-term follow-up is important given the potential for growth disturbances particularly with condylar fractures.

CLINICS CARE POINTS

- When working up a pediatric mandible fracture, perform a thorough clinical exam and appropriate radiographic exams including collateral information from guardians to identify potential fractures.
- Many pediatric mandible fractures can be treated with conservative management alone but require close follow-up.

- When choosing osteosynthesis plates for children undergoing open reduction internal fixation of a fracture, care should be taken to avoid critical structures, and hardware may warrant future removal.
- Children should have long term follow-up to evaluate for growth disturbances.

REFERENCES

1. Shahzad F. Pediatric Mandible Reconstruction: Controversies and Considerations. Plast Reconstr Surg Glob Open 2020;8:e3285.
2. Farkas LG, Posnick JC, Hreczko TM. Growth patterns of the face: a morphometric study. Cleft Palate Craniofac J 1992;29:308.
3. Mizoguchi I, Toriya N, Nakao Y. Growth of the mandible and biological characteristics of the mandibular condylar cartilage. Jpn Dent Sci Rev 2013;49:139.
4. Kaban LB, Mulliken JB, Murray JE. Facial fractures in children: an analysis of 122 fractures in 109 patients. Plast Reconstr Surg 1977;59:15.
5. Vyas RM, Dickinson BP, Wasson KL, et al. Pediatric facial fractures: current national incidence, distribution, and health care resource use. J Craniofac Surg 2008;19:339.
6. Hong K, Jeong J, Susson YN, et al. Patterns of pediatric facial fractures. Craniomaxillofacial Trauma Reconstr 2021;14:325.
7. Morisada MV, Tollefson TT, Said M, et al. Pediatric mandible fractures: mechanism, pattern of injury, fracture characteristics, and management by age. Facial Plast Surg Aesthet Med 2022;24:375.
8. Kao R, Rabbani CC, Patel JM, et al. Management of mandible fracture in 150 children across 7 years in a US tertiary care hospital. JAMA Facial Plast Surg 2019;21:414.
9. Hoppe IC, Kordahi AM, Paik AM, et al. Age and sex-related differences in 431 pediatric facial fractures at a level 1 trauma center. J Cranio-Maxillo-Fac Surg 2014;42:1408.
10. Cleveland CN, Kelly A, DeGiovanni J, et al. Maxillofacial trauma in children: association between age and mandibular fracture site. Am J Otolaryngol 2021;42:102874.
11. Iso-Kungas P, Törnwall J, Suominen AL, et al. Dental injuries in pediatric patients with facial fractures are frequent and severe. J Oral Maxillofac Surg 2012;70:396.
12. Owusu JA, Bellile E, Moyer JS, et al. Patterns of pediatric mandible fractures in the United States. JAMA Facial Plast Surg 2016;18:37.
13. Wheeler J, Phillips J. Pediatric facial fractures and potential long-term growth disturbances. Craniomaxillofacial Trauma Reconstr 2011;4:43.

14. Morris C, Kushner GM, Tiwana PS. Facial skeletal trauma in the growing patient. Oral Maxillofac Surg Clin 2012;24:351.

15. Smartt JM Jr, Low DW, Bartlett SP. The pediatric mandible: II. Management of traumatic injury or fracture. Plast Reconstr Surg 2005;116:28e.

16. Kannari L, Marttila E, Toivari M, et al. Paediatric mandibular fracture-a diagnostic challenge? Int J Oral Maxillofac Surg 2020;49:1439.

17. Ghosh R, Gopalkrishnan K, Anand J. Pediatric facial fractures: a 10-year study. J Maxillofac Oral Surg 2018;17:158.

18. Kannari L, Marttila E, Thorén H, et al. Dental injuries in paediatric mandibular fracture patients. Oral Maxillofac Surg 2022;26:99.

19. Major clinical considerations and treatment of mandible fracture: a concise systematic review. Int J Dev Res 2021;11(8):48723–7.

20. Nabaweesi R, Ramakrishnaiah RH, Aitken ME, et al. Injured children receive twice the radiation dose at nonpediatric trauma centers compared with pediatric trauma centers. J Am Coll Radiol 2018;15:58.

21. Kharbanda AB, Flood A, Blumberg K, et al. Analysis of radiation exposure among pediatric trauma patients at national trauma centers. J Trauma Acute Care Surg 2013;74:907.

22. Lindberg DM, Stence NV, Grubenhoff JA, et al. Feasibility and Accuracy of Fast MRI Versus CT for Traumatic Brain Injury in Young Children. Pediatrics 2019;144.

23. Feuerriegel GC, Ritschl LM, Sollmann N, et al. Imaging of traumatic mandibular fractures in young adults using CT-like MRI: a feasibility study. Clin Oral Investig 2023;27(3):1227–33.

24. Siy RW, Brown RH, Koshy JC, et al. General management considerations in pediatric facial fractures. J Craniofac Surg 2011;22:1190.

25. Posnick JC, Wells M, Pron GE. Pediatric facial fractures: evolving patterns of treatment. J Oral Maxillofac Surg 1993;51:836.

26. Pereira I, Pellizzer E, Lemos C, et al. Closed versus open reduction of facial fractures in children and adolescents: A systematic review and meta-analysis. J Clin Exp Dent 2021;13:e67.

27. Paggi Claus JD, Almeida MS, FDB dos S, et al. Pediatric bilateral condylar high displaced fracture: ten years follow-up. Craniomaxillofac Trauma Reconstr Open 2020;5. 2472751220944715.

28. Demianczuk AN, Verchere C, Phillips JH. The effect on facial growth of pediatric mandibular fractures. J Craniofac Surg 1999;10:323.

29. Goth S, Sawatari Y, Peleg M. Management of pediatric mandible fractures. J Craniofac Surg 2012;23:47.

30. Lopez J, Lake IV, Khavanin N, et al. Noninvasive management of pediatric isolated, condylar fractures: less is more? Plast Reconstr Surg 2021;147:443.

31. Stanton DC, Liu F, Yu JW, et al. Use of bioresorbable plating systems in paediatric mandible fractures. J Cranio-Maxillo-Fac Surg 2014;42:1305.

32. Bansal A, Yadav P, Bhutia O, et al. Comparison of outcome of open reduction and internal fixation versus closed treatment in pediatric mandible fractures-a retrospective study. J Cranio-Maxillo-Fac Surg 2021;49:196.

33. Madsen M, Tiwana PS, Alpert B. The use of risdon cables in pediatric maxillofacial trauma: a technique revisited. Craniomaxillofacial Trauma Reconstr 2012;5:107.

34. Aizenbud D, Hazan-Molina H, Emodi O, et al. The management of mandibular body fractures in young children. Dent Traumatol 2009;25:565.

35. Yadav S, Tyagi S, Kumar P, et al. Circummandibular wiring: an absolute answer to paediatric maxillofacial trauma: An unusual case report. SRM Journal of Research in Dental Sciences 2012;3:268.

36. Sharifi R, Hasheminasab M. The conservative treatment of pediatric mandible fracture with external nasal splint. J Craniofac Surg 2016;27:e562.

37. Boffano P, Roccia F, Schellino E, et al. Conservative treatment of unilateral displaced condylar fractures in children with mixed dentition. J Craniofac Surg 2012;23:e376.

38. Nørholt SE, Krishnan V, Sindet-Pedersen S, et al. Pediatric condylar fractures: a long-term follow-up study of 55 patients. J Oral Maxillofac Surg 1993;51:1302.

39. Zimmermann CE, Troulis MJ, Kaban LB. Pediatric facial fractures: recent advances in prevention, diagnosis and management. Int J Oral Maxillofac Surg 2005;34:823.

40. Yerit KC, Hainich S, Enislidis G, et al. Biodegradable fixation of mandibular fractures in children: stability and early results. Oral Surg Oral Med Oral Pathol Oral Radiol Endod 2005;100:17.

41. Singh M, Singh RK, Passi D, et al. Management of pediatric mandibular fractures using bioresorbable plating system - Efficacy, stability, and clinical outcomes: our experiences and literature review. J Oral Biol Craniofac Res 2016;6:101.

42. Pontell ME, Niklinska EB, Braun SA, et al. Resorbable versus titanium rigid fixation for pediatric mandibular fractures: a systematic review, institutional experience and comparative analysis. Craniomaxillofacial Trauma Reconstr 2022;15:189.

43. Posnick JC. Management of facial fractures in children and adolescents. Ann Plast Surg 1994;33:442.

44. Wolfswinkel EM, Weathers WM, Wirthlin JO, et al. Management of pediatric mandible fractures. Otolaryngol Clin North Am 2013;46:791.

45. Sharma S, Vashistha A, Chugh A, et al. Pediatric mandibular fractures: a review. Int J Clin Pediatr Dent 2009;2:1.

46. Yesantharao PS, Lopez J, Reategui A, et al. Open reduction, internal fixation of isolated mandible angle fractures in growing children. J Craniofac Surg 1946;31:2020.

47. Al-Moraissi EA, Ellis E 3rd. What method for management of unilateral mandibular angle fractures has the lowest rate of postoperative complications? A systematic review and meta-analysis. J Oral Maxillofac Surg 2014;72:2197.

48. Thorén H, Iizuka T, Hallikainen D, et al. An epidemiological study of patterns of condylar fractures in children. Br J Oral Maxillofac Surg 1997;35:306.

49. Lindahl L, Hollender L. Condylar fractures of the mandible. II. a radiographic study of remodeling processes in the temporomandibular joint. Int J Oral Surg 1977;6:153.

50. Steed MB, Schadel CM. Management of pediatric and adolescent condylar fractures. Atlas Oral Maxillofac Surg Clin North Am 2017;25:75.

51. Bae SS, Aronovich S. Trauma to the pediatric temporomandibular joint. Oral Maxillofac Surg Clin 2018; 30:47.

52. Tabrizi R, Langner NJ, Zamiri B, et al. Comparison of nonsurgical treatment options in pediatric condylar fractures: rigid intermaxillary fixation versus using guiding elastic therapy. J Craniofac Surg 2013;24: e203.

53. Dahlström L, Kahnberg KE, Lindahl L. 15 years follow-up on condylar fractures. Int J Oral Maxillofac Surg 1989;18:18.

54. Gilhuus-Moe O. Fractures of the mandibular condyle: a clinical and radiographic examination of 62 patients injured in the growth period. Trans Int Conf Oral Surg 1970;121.

55. Chang S, Yang Y, Liu Y, et al. How does the remodeling capacity of children affect the morphologic changes of fractured mandibular condylar processes after conservative treatment? J Oral Maxillofac Surg 2018;76:1279.e1.

56. Hovinga J, Boering G, Stegenga B. Long-term results of nonsurgical management of condylar fractures in children. Int J Oral Maxillofac Surg 1999; 28:429.

57. Dodson TB. Condyle and ramus-condyle unit fractures in growing patients: management and outcomes. Oral Maxillofac Surg Clin 2005;17:447.

58. Neff A, Chossegros C, Blanc J-L, et al., International Bone Research Association: Position paper from the IBRA Symposium on Surgery of the Head–the 2nd International Symposium for Condylar Fracture Osteosynthesis, Marseille, France 2012. J Craniomaxillofac Surg 42: 1234, 2014.

59. Lund K. Mandibular growth and remodelling processes after condylar fracture. A longitudinal roentgencephalometric study. Acta Odontol Scand Suppl 1974;32:3.

60. Posnick JC, Goldstein JA. Surgical management of temporomandibular joint ankylosis in the pediatric population. Plast Reconstr Surg 1993;91:791.

61. Laskin DM. Role of the meniscus in the etiology of posttraumatic temporomandibular joint ankylosis. Int J Oral Surg 1978;7:340.

62. Arakeri G, Kusanale A, Zaki GA, et al. Pathogenesis of post-traumatic ankylosis of the temporomandibular joint: a critical review. Br J Oral Maxillofac Surg 2012;50:8.

63. He D, Ellis E 3rd, Zhang Y. Etiology of temporomandibular joint ankylosis secondary to condylar fractures: the role of concomitant mandibular fractures. J Oral Maxillofac Surg 2008;66:77.

Pediatric Le Fort, Zygomatic, and Naso-Orbito-Ethmoid Fractures

Aparna Bhat, DMD, MD[a], Rachel Lim, DDS, MD[a], Mark A. Egbert, DDS[a,b,c], Srinivas M. Susarla, DMD, MD, MPH[a,b,c],*

KEYWORDS

- Le Fort fracture • Zygomaticomaxillary complex fracture • Naso-orbito-ethmoid fracture
- Pediatric facial trauma

KEY POINTS

- Fractures of the pediatric midface are relatively infrequent.
- Midface fracture patterns seen in children in the primary and mixed dentition are highly variable.
- Fracture patterns seen in adolescents and teenagers more closely resemble those seen in adults.
- Operative intervention should be considered for management of displaced fractures in children.
- Longitudinal follow-up to assess dental and facial development is critical.

INTRODUCTION

Pediatric facial fractures make up fewer than 15% of all facial fractures and comprise less than 5% of pediatric trauma admissions in the United States.[1] Midface fractures are not commonly seen in patients younger than 5 years of age.[2]

In infants, the cranium protrudes forward in comparison to the remaining bones of the face. Given the relative retrusion of the facial skeleton relative to the cranium, there is a much lower risk of facial fractures in infants and small children.[3,4] As children age, the craniofacial skeleton develops further, with downward and forward growth of the midface and mandible resulting in increased prominence of these portions of the face. At birth, the ratio of skull to face surface areas is projected to be about 8:1.[2–5] As the child develops, the ratio shifts until it reaches 2:1 in adulthood.[2,3] This change in ratio reflects the skull increasing to 4 times its original size, whereas the face increases to 12 times its original size.[3] The differential distribution of facial ratios in infants and young children relative to skeletally mature patients accounts for the difference in prevalence of facial fractures seen across these groups (**Figs. 1** and **2**). Although the nomenclature for midfacial fractures is consistent between children and adults (**Fig. 3**), the patterns of injury may be more variable in growing children (**Figs. 4–9**).

Anatomy

In comparison to the adult facial skeleton, children demonstrate increased bone pliability, unerupted teeth, incompletely developed sinuses and a thicker layer of subcutaneous fat.[3–6] These factors render children more likely to absorb greater energy transfers without sustaining displaced facial fractures.[6] The lack of a fully developed frontal sinus results in less potential for shock absorption from blunt force trauma. This, in turn, allows for the frontal force to be transmitted to the supraorbital bar, basilar, skull and intracranially. Beginning

[a] Department of Oral and Maxillofacial Surgery, University of Washington School of Dentistry, 1959 NE Pacific Street, B-307, Seattle, WA 98195, USA; [b] Department of Surgery, Division of Plastic Surgery, University of Washington School of Medicine, 1959 NE Pacific Street, B-307, Seattle, WA 98195, USA; [c] Craniofacial Center, Seattle Children's Hospital, 4800 Sand Point Way NE, Seattle, WA 98015, USA
* Corresponding author. Department of Oral and Maxillofacial Surgery, University of Washington School of Dentistry, University of Washington, Seattle, WA.
E-mail address: Srinivas.susarla@seattlechildrens.org

Oral Maxillofacial Surg Clin N Am 35 (2023) 563–575
https://doi.org/10.1016/j.coms.2023.04.004
1042-3699/23/

REGION		% GROWTH COMPLETED BY AGE 1	% GROWTH COMPLETED BY AGE 5	SKELETAL MATURITY
Upper Face	Cranial Vault	84–85	90–94	14–16 y
	Orbits	85	88–93	Variable
Midface	Zygoma	72	83	13–15 years
	Maxilla	75–80	85	14–15 years
Lower Face	Mandible	60–70	74–85	14–16+ years

Fig. 1. The various regions of the face complete growth at different ages. Cranial vault (upper face) has nearly completed growth as patients transition from the primary dentition to the mixed dentition. In contrast, midface growth continues over the mixed dentition, nearing completion as patients transition to the permanent dentition.

at 2 years of age, the ethmoid and maxillary sinuses begin to enlarge, and the sphenoid and frontal sinuses begin to appear.[4] The sinuses continue to grow, reaching full size after adolescence. As the sinuses develop, the bone of the midface begins to thin, providing decreased resistance to fracture when compared to infancy.[4] Additionally, the flexible nature of pediatric bones gives children a greater likelihood of sustaining greenstick fractures.[3,6] As children approach skeletal maturity, the differences between pediatric and adult facial skeletons are minimal.[4]

Common Etiologies

Children are less apt to sustain serious midface trauma with blunt force frontal impact, given their

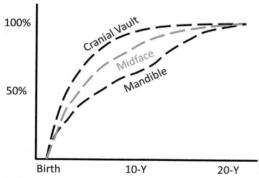

Fig. 2. Growth velocity of the cranial vault (upper face) relative to the midface and mandible (lower face). In contrast to cranial vault growth, which occurs rapidly in the first few years of life, midface growth velocity tapers in the mixed dentition, leveling off as patients reach the permanent dentition.

anatomy. Midface fracture patterns in infants and small children are typically the result of high-energy transfer mechanisms, such as motor vehicle accidents.[7] As children grow, fracture etiologies begin to more closely resemble those in adults: motor vehicle accidents, sports, and assault.[8]

Initial Evaluation

As with any trauma patient, adherence to Advanced Trauma Life Support (ATLS) principles is paramount in the evaluation of the injured child.[9,10] One should ensure that the patient's airway is evaluated and free of any obstructions. Additionally, the patient's cervical spine should be assessed, and patient should remain in a rigid collar to allow for stabilization until cervical spine injury can be ruled out. Given that pediatric midface fractures are typically seen in cases with high velocity impact, patients may be intubated upon arrival to the hospital. However, if this is not the case, upon initial assessment, the airway should be immediately evaluated. If the patient is unable to maintain their airway independently, orotracheal intubation should be considered. If orotracheal intubation is unable to be achieved, one can consider cricothyroidotomy in an emergency setting. If an obstruction is present to the lower airway, an emergency tracheostomy can be considered. Once an airway is definitively established, primary survey per ATLS protocol should be completed.

Evaluation of the facial skeleton remains a part of the secondary survey after airway, breathing, circulation, disability, and exposure are addressed. Patients with midface trauma will benefit not only from evaluation by the maxillofacial trauma surgeon, but also from evaluations by Ophthalmology to rule out

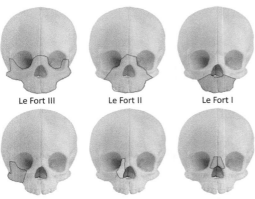

Le Fort III   Le Fort II   Le Fort I

Zygomaticomaxillary   Naso-Orbito-Ethmoid   Nasal Bone
Complex

Fig. 3. Facial fracture patterns seen in adults can occur in pediatric patients, but may be more variable in presentation. However, the nomenclature for the patterns of injury remains the same.

ocular injury in patients with fractures involving the orbit (Le Fort II, Le Fort III, zygomaticomaxillary complex [ZMC], and naso-orbito-ethmoid [NOE]) and neurosurgery if skull fractures or intracranial injury is evident or suspected.

Treatment Considerations: General Principles

Management of pediatric facial injuries requires an understanding of the natural growth and

development of the facial skeleton. Although the goals of treatment of displaced facial fractures are the same as in adults, reduction into anatomic alignment and immobilization to allow for fracture healing, the methods by which these are achieved may need to be modified. Surgical exposures should be tailored to minimize subperiosteal dissection to only that needed to visualize the fracture and, if needed, apply fixation. When considering fixation, both titanium and resorbable fixation may be considered appropriate in contemporary practice. Fixation should be placed with recognition of the location of succcedaneous teeth (**Fig. 10**). Titanium fixation may afford the opportunity for greater rigidity with lower profile plates, but comes at the cost of the need for removal after bony healing in growing patients. Resorbable fixation devices have become more popular in this context, but may be less rigid and require thicker fixation plates.[11–14] However, as children have much more robust healing than adults, the paradigms for rigid fixation of the adult facial skeleton may not apply to children. Less rigid fixation may result in sufficient immobilization to allow for bony union.[15]

Timing of repair is challenging given the quick healing nature of pediatric tissues. Ideally, one should pursue operative management within 1 week of injury, with some authors suggesting repair as soon as 2 to 4 days after injury.[16]

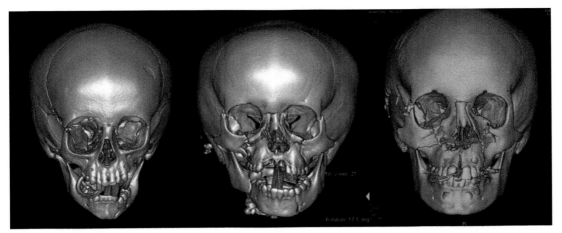

Fig. 4. Maxillary fractures at the various Le Fort levels are uncommon in children, but may present in the context of high-energy mechanisms. In young patients, incomplete, nondisplaced injuries are more likely, due to the lack of aerated sinuses and relative retrusion of the midface relative to the upper face. As the midface develops with anterior and inferior growth, Le Fort fracture patterns become more consistent with those seen in adults. High-energy mechanisms may result in comminuted fractures of the midface in isolation, or as a component of a panfacial injury. (*Left*) Non-displaced bilateral Le Fort III fracture in a 2 year old patient with an associated non-displaced left mandibular parasymphyseal fracture. (*Middle*) Comminuted midface injury with multi-level Le Fort injuries in a patient in the early mixed dentition. (*Right*) Isolated, multi-level Le Fort fractures in a patient in the later mixed dentition.

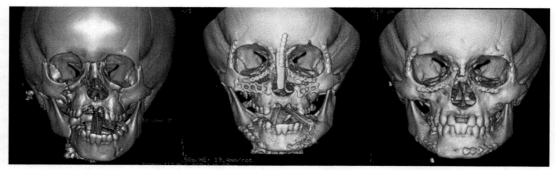

Fig. 5. In this patient with multi-level Le Fort injuries (*Left*), open reduction and internal fixation of the midface was performed via coronal, lower eyelid, and maxillary vestibular approaches; the nasal dorsum was reconstructed with a cantilever cranial bone graft (*Middle*). Rigid fixation was achieved with titanium miniplates. Miniplates on the lower midface were removed shortly after confirmation of bony healing, to facilitate dentoalveolar development (*Right*).

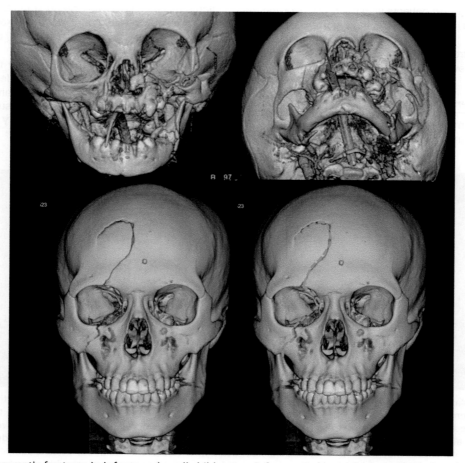

Fig. 6. Zygomatic fractures in infants and small children are infrequent, due to the lack of developed maxillary sinuses. High-energy mechanisms can result in comminuted injuries (*top*, 1 year old infant with comminuted zygomatic injury from dog bite) or unusual fracture patterns (*bottom*, 12 year old patient with incomplete zygomatic fracture propagating through the orbit into the frontal bone).

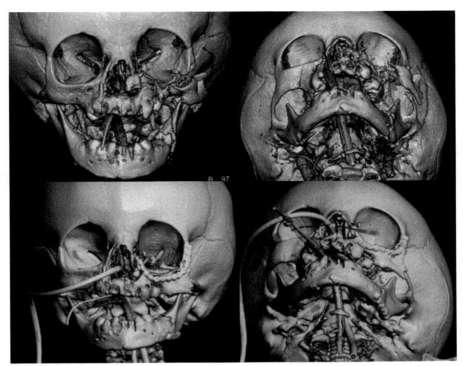

Fig. 7. Management of comminuted injuries in small children frequently requires the use of autologous bone grafts. In this patient, the comminuted left zygomaticomaxillary complex and orbital floor (*top*) were reconstructed using calvarial bone graft (*bottom*).

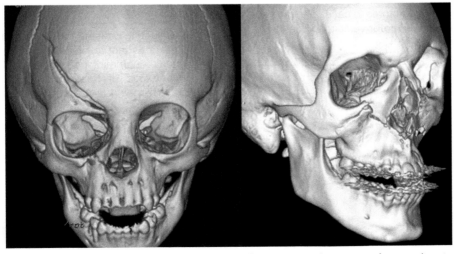

Fig. 8. (*Left*) In patients in the primary dentition, the lack of large aerated sinuses and a prominent cranium results in a low frequency of midface fractures. High-energy transfers typically cause nondisplaced midface injuries, but associated skull fractures, as seen in this 2 year old patient. (*Right*) In patients in the permanent dentition, midface fracture patterns more closely resemble those in adult patients, as seen in this 14 year old patient with a type I naso-orbito-ethmoid fracture.

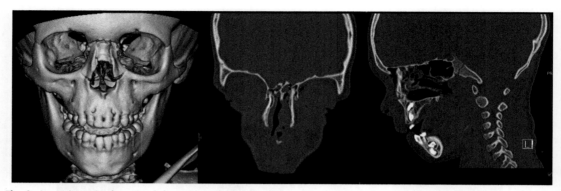

Fig. 9. In patients in the mixed dentition, displaced midface fractures may be more likely to occur, with posterior and superior displacement, as seen in this 6 year old patient with displaced bilateral NOE fracures impacted into the anterior skull base.

LE FORT FRACTURES
Anatomy

The classic Le Fort fracture patterns as described by Rene Le Fort in 1901 are less commonly seen in children given the relative pliability of pediatric skeletal structure when compared to that of adults (see **Figs. 4** and **5**). In general, Le Fort fracture patterns are rarely seen in children under the age of 6 years.[2] Previous studies have reported that children with mixed or solely primary dentition do not sustain Le Fort type fractures. However, this notion has been disputed by some authors who have noted equal distribution of Le Fort type fractures among children with primary, mixed, secondary dentition.[2] In general, the likelihood of sustaining a Le Fort type fracture pattern is greater in older children compared to infants and young children. Pediatric patients most commonly sustain Le Fort type fractures in cases of high velocity impact, such as in motor vehicle accidents.[2,6,17]

Classification

A common component of all Le Fort fractures is disruption of the pterygomaxillary junction. The Le Fort I fracture pattern results from a horizontal force delivered to the level of the patient's dentition. The Le Fort I fracture pattern involves separation of the lower midface (maxilla and alveolus) from the zygoma and nasal complex, as the fracture extends laterally from the zygomaticomaxillary buttress to the nasomaxillary buttress at the level of the piriform rim. The Le Fort II fracture ("pyramidal fracture") pattern extends from the nasofrontal suture down through the zygomaticomaxillary suture, with the resultant fractured segment resembling a pyramidal structure. The Le Fort III fracture ("craniofacial disjunction") pattern is noted to produce a convex or dish-shaped facial deformity. It extends from the nasofrontal suture through the floor of the orbit, and fractures at the lateral orbital rim, and zygomatic arch.

Clinical Examination

When evaluating patients for Le Fort fracture patterns, it is important to evaluate for potential hemorrhage, although midface trauma is unlikely to be the sole cause of hemodynamic instability. If persistent bleeding is present, the region should

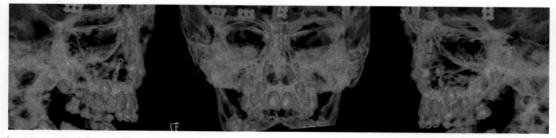

Fig. 10. Internal fixation for displaced midface fractures can utilize titanium fixation or resorbable fixation. Titanium fixation allows for greater rigidity for a given plate thickness, but may need to be removed when placed in the growing skeleton. Regardless of the type of fixation, extreme care should be taken to avoid injury to succedaneous dentition when placing fixation along the nasomaxillary and zygomaticomaxillary buttresses. Monocortical fixation with short screw lengths is paramount.

be packed if immediate control of the vessel is unable to be achieved. Continued hemorrhage that is unable to be controlled with packing may warrant operative exploration or angiography and embolization. Once bleeding is controlled, the provider should perform a thorough facial examination.

One should take note of any external lacerations present, document the depth of injury and involved tissues. Any obvious depression or displacement of the patient's skeletal structure is suggestive of displaced facial bone injury. Patterns of ecchymoses may correspond with particular injuries, such as postauricular ecchymoses with skull base fractures (Battle's sign), periorbital ecchymoses with NOE fractures, and palatal/mucosal ecchymoses with maxillary fractures (Guerin's sign). Next, assess for bleeding or drainage from the patients ears and nose. If clear drainage is noted within either the ear canal or nose, cerebrospinal fluid (CSF) leak should be suspected, and neurosurgical evaluation requested. The patient should also be asked if they have a metallic or salty taste, as this can be another indication of a CSF leak. Intranasal examination should include assessment of bleeding, septal deviation, or hematoma.

One should then systematically palpate the bones of the face starting from top to bottom to assess for any step offs. Palpate the superior rims of the orbits, followed by the lateral rims, the inferior rims, nasal bones, and zygomas. Next, assess for any mobility of the maxilla by placing the index finger on the anterior palate and the thumb within the labial vestibule and pulling inferiorly, anteriorly, and laterally. The provider should assess intraorally for any lacerations, displaced teeth, or region of ecchymosis.

Management

Management of pediatric Le Fort type fractures is debated, though most clinicians favor early surgical repair for displaced fractures. Operative management is typically pursued as these fractures tend to have more complicated fracture patterns given the mechanism of injury. However, some authors argue that given the increased osteogenic potential of the pediatric skeleton, many facial fractures can be managed conservatively when compared with their adult counterparts.[15] Ultimately, most providers tend to treat Le Fort type I fracture patterns operatively.[4,17]

Regardless of the level of the Le Fort injury, management will frequently include reduction of the occlusal unit and application of intermaxillary fixation. Intermaxillary fixation in children may be challenging due to the incomplete eruption of teeth, interdental spacing, and variable stability

of primary teeth in the mixed dentition. The use of intermaxillary fixation screws or related appliances is strictly contraindicated in patients in the primary dentition and those in the mixed dentition in regions where the permanent teeth have not erupted.

Surgical approaches to Le Fort I fracture in children are similar to those in adults. Access to the nasomaxillary and zygomaticomaxillary buttresses is readily achieved via a maxillary vestibular approach. Patients with Le Fort II pattern injuries may require additional exposures of the infraorbital rim and/or nasofrontal junction. In isolated Le Fort II injuries, local incisions are suitable for accessing these areas. In patients with concomitant upper face injuries, a coronal exposure may be indicated. In addition to the exposures utilized for the central midface in Le Fort II fractures, exposure of the lateral orbital wall via upper eyelid approaches and zygomatic arch via a coronal approach, may be indicated in patients with Le Fort III injuries.

ZYGOMATICOMAXILLARY COMPLEX FRACTURES
Anatomy

Zygomaticomaxillary complex (ZMC) fractures are the most common fracture patterns associated with high impact traumas in children, with 15% of pediatric facial fractures being attributed to ZMC fractures (see **Figs. 6** and **7**).[1] The next most common fracture patterns are maxillary dentoalveolar fractures, and nasal bone fractures.[18] The anatomy of the ZMC involves the zygoma, the maxilla, and the orbital floor. The lack of pneumatization and the thicker walls of the pediatric sinuses allow for extra support to the zygomatic buttress, thereby producing an area of increased resistance to fracture. The increased cancellous-to-cortical bone ratio and flexibility at the suture lines provides another layer of protection to the ZMC region. As children age, the sinuses begin to develop, and the increased aeration to the maxillary sinuses, in addition to the eruption of the secondary dentition, causes growth of the midface and mandible, leaving the midface more vulnerable to fracture. In children, isolated zygomatic fractures rarely are seen as the bones surrounding the zygoma are very thin. The zygoma acts as a horizontal buttress, and with high velocity impact, will distribute the force to the adjacent bones, thereby resulting in concomitant fractures to the NOE complex, the orbit, and the skull.

Clinical Examination

The clinical examination for patients with suspected ZMC fracture patterns should start by evaluating for any obvious facial deformity to the malar eminences. One should make sure to evaluate from the superior, inferior, frontal, and lateral views to best assess for any displacement. The superior view is the best view to evaluate posterior displacement of the zygoma and potential for facial flattening. Next the provider should palpate starting at the medial portion of the inferior orbital rim, moving laterally toward the zygomatic arch, over the malar eminences, down toward the maxilla. As the ZMC involves the maxilla, it is also important to inspect and palpate intraorally, in the region of the buccal vestibule to assess for any regions of ecchymosis or dentoalveolar fractures, respectively.

Given that the orbital floor is typically involved in the fracture line, a thorough eye examination should be performed. Findings such as diplopia, unequal pupillary levels, enophthalmos, inferior displacement of the palpebral ligament, and subconjunctival hemorrhage may be seen. During the examination, the provider should also assess for full extraocular movements to ensure no signs of muscle entrapment. If full movements are not noted initially, one must perform a forced duction test to confirm restricted ocular movement. If there are any concerns during the eye examination, ophthalmology should be consulted for further evaluation. As the infraorbital nerve is often involved with these injuries, one may expect to find some degree of paresthesia present to the infraorbital region, maxilla and around the nose.

It is not uncommon to note periorbital ecchymosis, and as such it is also important to concurrently inspect for Battle's sign by assessing behind the patient's ears to note any hint of basilar skull fracture. If the zygoma is posteriorly displaced, one may note flattening of the malar eminences which can be best assessed from the superior view. The presence of edema may cause difficulties in assessment of malar positioning. Trismus may be seen in some patients as the zygoma may be displaced medially, thereby causing a physical stop for full opening of the mandible. As with any clinical exam, the provider should utilize radiographic imaging, specifically CT imaging, to create a complete inventory of the patient's injuries.

Management

Management of ZMC fractures is divided as clinicians prefer to utilize conservative nonsurgical measures in pediatric populations so as not to disrupt midface and dental development.[18] However, as ZMC fractures are typically seen with high velocity impact injuries, which also tend to produce more comminuted or displaced fractures, open reduction and internal fixation (ORIF) is often required to prevent future growth disturbances.[18,19]

ORIF with miniplates and screws has become the standard of care for management of displaced ZMC fractures. During surgery, the surgeon must first ensure reduction of the spheno-zygomatic suture, as this allows for a more precise reconstruction with better aesthetic results. As with adult ZMC reconstruction, one must then ensure reduction of zygomaticofrontal suture, and the infraorbital rim, to ensure proper reduction before proceeding with fixation. The need for 1-, 2-, or 3-point fixation for adequate fixation will vary depending upon the degree of comminution and location of the fracture.[18,19]

Surgical intervention should ideally be performed within 3 to 5 days after initial edema has resolved to avoid improper healing which may require reoperation.[18] When performing exposure of the infraorbital rim through transconjunctival or transcutaneous approaches, it is paramount to resuspend the soft tissues of the midface to the rim following bony reduction. Failure to do so will frequently result in midface soft tissue ptosis and premature aging, as well as potentially contribute to lower eyelid malposition (ectropion).

NASO-ORBITO-ETHMOID FRACTURES
Anatomy

NOE fracture patterns involve the superior portion of the midface, specifically the nasal bones, the frontal bones, portions of the medial, superior and inferior orbital walls, and the ethmoid bones (see **Figs. 8–10**; **Figs. 11–13**). These fracture patterns in children are also typically only seen with high-speed velocity impact, such as in motor vehicle accidents, and tend to comprise less than 1% of pediatric facial fractures.[12,20] The NOE region is important as it is the physical junction between the forehead, nose, orbits, and upper midface.[21] Injury to this area and subsequent operative treatment can make subsequent growth difficult to predict. With NOE fractures, the age of the child heavily influences fracture patterns, especially as children younger than 2 years old tend to have more flexible bones, leading to greater potential for greenstick fractures. It is also important to note that while the ethmoid, maxillary, and frontal sinuses are all present at birth, the frontal sinus only starts to develop when children are around 4 to 5 years of age. The lack of a fully developed frontal sinus leads to less potential for shock absorption from blunt force trauma.[21] This can result in force being directed into the supraorbital region and skull

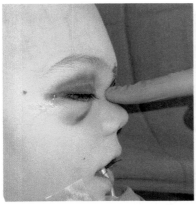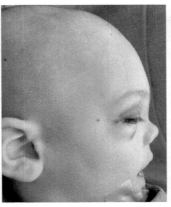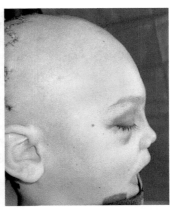

Fig. 11. Disruption of the naso-orbito-ethmoid complex in children is typically associated with posterior and superior displacement (*left*). Loss of support to the nasal dorsum results in a saddle nose deformity (*middle*) that, if uncorrected acutely, poses a significant reconstructive challenge in the future. Acute reconstruction typically requires reduction and fixation of the NOE segments as well as dorsal nasal reconstruction with cantileveler bone graft (*right*).

base. For this reason, it is of utmost importance to consider intracranial hemorrhage and dural injury with associated CSF leak, especially in children who present with NOE fractures and basilar skull fractures.[21]

Classification

Although several different classification systems have arisen to describe different types of NOE fractures, the most commonly used is that derived by Manson and Markowitz in 1991. This scheme defines 3 types of NOE fractures, based on attachment of the medial canthal tendon (MCT) and the presence comminution of the fractured bone. Type I NOE fractures are described as those in which the MCT remains attached to a large, noncomminuted fragment. A type II NOE fracture is described as a fracture in which the MCT remains attached to bone; however, the region of fracture is comminuted. Type III NOE fractures are the most complex

fracture patterns, wherein the degree of comminution is severe, to the extent that the MCT is avulsed from its bony attachment.

Although the Markowitz system works well to classify adult NOE fractures, it does not always describe the fracture patterns sustained by children. This is most likely because it does not account for the differences in pediatric anatomy such as the proportions of the craniofacial skeleton in children and the lack of pneumatization of the sinuses.[21] As such, the Burstein classification was created to better describe the NOE fracture patterns sustained by children. A Burstein type I NOE fracture pattern is a unilateral fracture involving the portion of frontal bone medial to the superior orbital foramen as well as the superior portion of the NOE complex. A Burstein type II NOE fracture pattern is also unilateral in nature, involving the superior orbital rim and extending halfway up the frontal bone. A Burstein type III NOE fracture pattern is bilateral, includes the

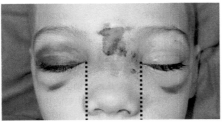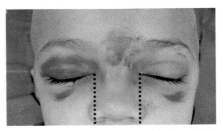

Fig. 12. Displaced naso-orbito-ethmoid fractures in small children will often result in widening of the intercanthal distance (*left*). Assessing the integrity of the medial canthal tendon attachment, as in adults, is critical for determining the appropriate operative approach. In type I and type II injuries, anatomic reduction of the NOE segments typically results in improvement of the intercanthal distance (*right*). Medial canthoplasty is indicated in patients with comminuted injuries resulting in avulsion of the tendon from its bony attachments.

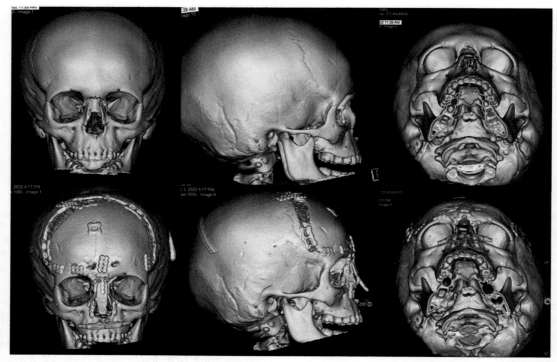

Fig. 13. Posteriorly and superiorly displaced bilateral type I naso-orbito-ethmoid fractures in a 6 year old child (*top row*). The NOE fractures were displaced through the anterior skull base, resulting in a large fronto-basilar defect with associated CSF leak. Open reduction and internal fixation was undertaken to address the skull base defect, CSF leak, and correct the central nasal projection. The nasal dorsum was reconstructed with a cantilever cranial bone graft. Postoperative images (*bottom row*) show reconstitution of the dorsal nasal project and correction of the NOE complex sagittal and vertical position.

superior orbital rims and the superior portion of the NOE complex, and involves the frontal bone.[21]

Clinical Examination

When performing clinical examination for patients with suspected NOE fractures, findings may include telecanthus, retrusion of the nose at the nasofrontal region, or enophthalmos. Given that patients with medial orbital rim fractures are more likely to develop enophthalmos, it is particularly important to identify this risk, and assess any discrepancies during examination. Additionally, given the propensity for frontal forces to be directed to the supraorbital bar and skull base, one must consider the possibility of intracranial hemorrhage or dural injury with associated CSF leak. Postauricular ecchymoses may be suggestive of skull base injury; periorbital ecchymoses ("racoon eyes") may suggest NOE injury.

To examine the attachment of the MCT, one should place 2 fingers of one hand to traverse the bridge of the nose, whereas using the other hand to pull laterally next to the lateral canthus.

One may appreciate a positive bowstring sign if the MCT displaces laterally with this maneuver, indicating involvement of the MCT within the fracture. The hand that is bridging the nasal bridge may be able to feel if the fracture segments are comminuted or large and intact.

Another maneuver to assess the MCT is placement of a straight instrument such as a Freer elevator within the nose to the level of the MCT. With the other hand, the provider can palpate the region of the MCT externally. By manipulating the instrument, one can appreciate the state of the MCT with respect to its bony attachment.

One should also examine for telecanthus by measuring both the intercanthal distance and the interpupillary distance. As the nasal bones are typically affected, it is important to perform a thorough intranasal examination, and inspect for signs of nasal septal hematoma and intranasal bleeding. Lastly, given the proximity of the lacrimal duct to this area, it is important to thoroughly examine the duct to ensure patency. If the lacrimal duct is involved within the injury, an ophthalmology consult is recommended.

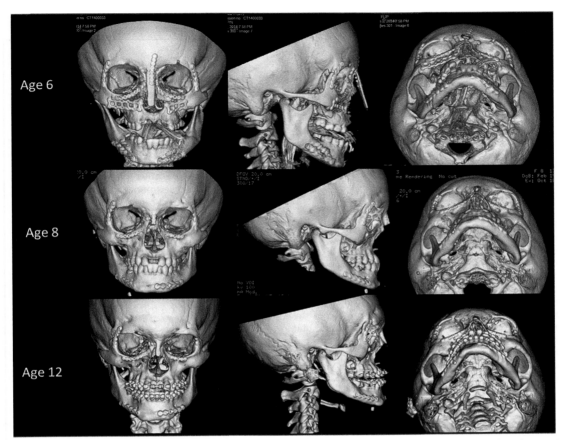

Age 6

Age 8

Age 12

Fig. 14. For severe injuries, such as panfacial fractures, rigid fixation is required to address displaced and comminuted injuries. This patient sustained panfacial injuries secondary to a motor vehicle accident at age 6 years. They were treated with open reduction and placement of titanium fixation across the midface buttresses, as well as the mandible. After a period of initial healing, the lower midface and tension band fixation in the mandible was removed. At age 8 years, there has been continued growth of the midface and mandible. At age 12 years, there is evolving maxillomandibular discrepancy, which will likely need to be addressed with orthognathic surgery at skeletal maturity. The cantilever nasal bone graft placed at the time of intervention has largely resorbed at the nasal tip, but the nasal radix morphology is preserved.

Management

The goals of NOE fracture management are to: restore intercanthal distance, correct positioning of the orbit, provide dorsal nasal support, and to preserve nasal tip projection. As discussed previously, the main anatomic areas that need to be addressed are the MCT, orbital rims, nasal bones, and potentially the nasal septum.

The repair of a Markowitz type I NOE fracture typically requires superior and inferior fixation to return the MCT to its proper positioning. If the orbital floor is involved, this can be reconstructed with calvarial bone graft or mesh (resorbable or titanium).

The repair of Markowitz type II and type III NOE fractures is more complex, as full exposure of the MCT is often required given the degree of comminution of the bony attachments or lack thereof.[22] Full exposure also will allow for proper bony reduction and canthal reinsertion. For proper stabilization, transnasal wiring is often recommended to provide accurate positioning of the bilateral MCT with respect to one another. To do so, one must ensure posterior placement of the transnasal wiring, as anterior placement of the wire will result in telecanthus due to medial displacement of the anterior bone. This displacement will result in lateral flaring of the posterior segments that constitute the medial orbital wall.

Multiple authors have advocated for using lead plates with felt lining for postoperative splint.[21] This assists both with soft tissue contouring and provides added force to medialize the canthal tendons. The addition of felt lining helps to prevent soft tissue erosion.

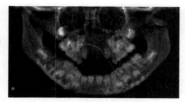

Post-Injury ORIF
(Age 6)

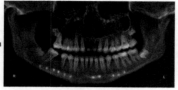

Permanent Dentition
(Age 13)

Fig. 15. Successful dental eruption following open reduction of multiple facial fractures. This 6 year old child underwent open reduction and internal fixation of bilateral orbital floor, ZMC, NOE, and mandibular fractures. The primary and permanent maxillary central incisors and right mandibular first permanent molar were lost at the time of the injury. In the early mixed dentition, there is appropriate eruption of the remaining permanent maxillary incisors, mandibular incisors, and first molars. At age 13 years, there has been complete eruption of the remaining succedaneous teeth. Note the remodeling of the left condyle, which was treated in a closed manner.

Additionally, it is important to consider that the bones of the nose and the medial orbital rims are relatively thin and fragile, and with NOE fractures, one can see collapse of the ethmoid bones, disruption of the nasal septum, as well as blunting of the nasal dorsal projection ("saddle nose deformity"). As such it is important to consider this during reconstruction. One should consider the use of bone and cartilage for grafting materials to reestablish the structure and support of the NOE region. Restoration of the nasal height and length, specifically, will most likely require placement of a cantilever bone graft. This can be achieved by using cranial bone, rib, or rib with a distal cartilage tip. The graft can easily be secured via miniplate fixation to the nasofrontal region. The bone graft should be positioned such that it caudally supports the tip. One can seek to address lacrimal duct injury; however, this is not typically performed at the time of primary surgery due to the relative difficulty of cannulation of the lacrimal duct.

FUNDING

The work was supported, in part, by the University of Washington Department of Oral and Maxillofacial Surgery Education and Research Fund.

CLINICS CARE POINTS

- Midface injuries in infants and small children are relatively infrequent, due to the retruded position of the midface relative to the upper face. When injuries occur, they are typically nondisplaced and can frequently be managed nonoperatively.

- Displaced midfacial fractures are seen most often in the context of high-energy transfers and require operative management to reduce the fractured segments into anatomic alignment. Failure to reduce displaced midfacial fractures, particularly those involving the external orbital framework (ZMC, NOE, Le Fort II–III) may result in complex midface deformities that are difficult to address with secondary corrective osteotomies.[18,23]

- The tenets of surgical repair are to minimize subperiosteal stripping, achieve anatomic alignment of the fractured segments, and use the least amount of fixation necessary to allow for bony healing. Following confirmation of bony healing, patients will still need to be followed closely over time (**Figs. 14** and **15**), as traumatic disruptions of growth centers may result in secondary deformities, even following appropriate surgical management.[23]

- At skeletal maturity, patients with midface injuries may have midface retrusion necessitating orthodontic or surgical management of malocclusion, asymmetry, or soft tissue deficiencies.[2,24–26]

REFERENCES

1. Imahara SD, Hopper RA, Wang J, et al. Patterns and outcomes of pediatric facial fractures in the United States: a survey of the National Trauma Data Bank. J Am Coll Surg 2008;207(5):710–6.

2. Macmillan A, Lopez J, Luck JD, et al. How Do Le Fort-Type Fractures Present in a Pediatric Cohort? J Oral Maxillofac Surg 2018;76(5):1044–54.

3. Mukherjee CG, Mukherjee U. Maxillofacial Trauma in Children. Int J Clin Pediatr Dent 2012;5(3):231–6.

4. Yu J, Dinsmore R, Mar P, et al. Pediatric maxillary fractures. J Craniofac Surg 2011;22(4):1247–50.

5. Zimmermann CE, Troulis MJ, Kaban LB. Pediatric facial fractures: recent advances in prevention, diagnosis and management. Int J Oral Maxillofac Surg 2006;35(1):2–13.

6. Dalena MM, Khan W, Dobitsch AA, et al. Patterns of Le Fort Fractures in the Pediatric Population. Am Surg 2019;85(8):408–10.

7. Yazici A, Aytaç I. Pediatric Maxillofacial Trauma Patterns Among Different Types of Road Traffic Accidents. J Craniofac Surg 2019;30(7):2039–41.

8. Kao R, Campiti VJ, Rabbani CC, et al. Pediatric Midface Fractures: Outcomes and Complications of 218 Patients. Laryngoscope Investig Otolaryngol 2019; 4(6):597–601.

9. Rogan DT, Ahmed A. Pediatric Facial Fractures. 2022. In: StatPearls [Internet]. Treasure Island (FL). StatPearls Publishing; 2023.

10. Andrew TW, Morbia R, Lorenz HP. Pediatric Facial Trauma. Clin Plast Surg 2019;46(2):239–47.

11. Rodriguez-Feliz J, Mehta K, Patel A. The management of pediatric type 1 nasoorbitoethmoidal fractures with resorbable fixation. J Craniofac Surg 2014;25(5):495–501.

12. Le TT, Berlin RS, Oleck NC, et al. Patterns of Nasoorbitalethmoid Fractures in the Pediatric Population. Am Surg 2019;85(7):730–2.

13. Eppley BL. Use of resorbable plates and screws in pediatric facial fractures. J Oral Maxillofac Surg 2005;63(3):385–91.

14. Triana RJ Jr, Shockley WW. Pediatric zygomatico-orbital complex fractures: the use of resorbable plating systems. A case report. J Craniomaxillofac Trauma 1998;4(4):32–6.

15. Chandra SR, Zemplenyi KS. Issues in Pediatric Craniofacial Trauma. Facial Plast Surg Clin North Am 2017;25(4):581–91.

16. Haug RH, Foss J. Maxillofacial injuries in the pediatric patient. Oral Surg Oral Med Oral Pathol Oral Radiol Endod 2000;90:126–34.

17. Moffitt JK, Cepeda A Jr, Wainwright DJ, et al. The Epidemiology and Management of Pediatric Maxillary Fractures. J Craniofac Surg 2021;32(3):859–62.

18. DeFazio MV, Fan KL, Avashia YJ, et al. Fractures of the pediatric zygoma: a review of the clinical trends, management strategies, and outcomes associated with zygomatic fractures in children. J Craniofac Surg 2013;24(6):1891–7.

19. Luck JD, Lopez J, Faateh M, et al. Pediatric Zygomaticomaxillary Complex Fracture Repair: Location and Number of Fixation Sites in Growing Children. Plast Reconstr Surg 2018;142(1):51e–60e.

20. Luthringer MM, Oleck NC, Mukherjee TJ, et al. Management of Pediatric Nasoorbitoethmoid Complex Fractures at a Level 1 Trauma Center. Am Surg 2022;88(7):1675–9.

21. Liau JY, Woodlief J, van Aalst JA. Pediatric nasoorbitoethmoid fractures. J Craniofac Surg 2011;22(5):1834–8.

22. Lopez J, Luck JD, Faateh M, et al. Pediatric Nasoorbitoethmoid Fractures: Cause, Classification, and Management. Plast Reconstr Surg 2019;143(1):211–22.

23. Yesantharao PS, Lopez J, Chang A, et al. The Association of Zygomaticomaxillary Complex Fractures with Naso-Orbitoethmoid Fractures in Pediatric Populations. Plast Reconstr Surg 2021;147(5):777e–86e.

24. Davidson EH, Schuster L, Rottgers SA, et al. Severe Pediatric Midface Trauma: A Prospective Study of Growth and Development. J Craniofac Surg 2015; 26(5):1523–8.

25. Schliephake H, Berten JL, Neukam FW, et al. Growth disorders following fractures of the midface in children. Dtsch Zahnarztl Z 1990;45(12):819–22.

26. Singh DJ, Bartlett SP. Pediatric craniofacial fractures: long-term consequences. Clin Plast Surg 2004;31:499–518.

Pediatric Nasal and Septal Fractures

Philip D. Tolley, MD[a,b], Benjamin B. Massenburg, MD[a,b], Scott Manning, MD[a,c], G. Nina Lu, MD[c], Randall A. Bly, MD[a,c],*

KEYWORDS

- Pediatric • Nasal fracture • Septal fracture • Craniofacial trauma • Fracture management

KEY POINTS

- Pediatric nasal fractures are less common in younger children but become increasingly more prevalent with age and comprise nearly one-third of all pediatric facial fractures.
- The nasal septum is an important growth center for nasal/midface development and disturbances in potential future growth are considered when determining a treatment plan.
- Immediate intervention for complications such as septal hematoma is critical to prevent abscess formation, septal perforation, or other late/delayed deformities later in life.
- The majority of pediatric nasoseptal fractures can be managed with closed reduction and splinting.
- Formal open septorhinoplasty at skeletal maturity is an important aspect of treatment of pediatric nasal bone fractures because many patients develop or have persistent nasal deformity/dysfunction even after closed reduction.

INTRODUCTION

Although craniofacial trauma in the pediatric population is less common than in adults, it still accounts for approximately 11% of all pediatric emergency room visits.[1] Although less common than in the adult population, nasal bone fractures make up close to one-third of these visits, making them similarly one of the most injured structures in the facial skeleton.[2] This may also underrepresent the true incidence as often when fractures do occur, unless severely displaced, parents do not seek medical intervention and fractures heal spontaneously.[3] Previous studies have shown that fractures predominantly occur in men and the frequency of injury increases as children grow closer to adulthood.[4,5] As children age, the causes of nasal fractures also change beginning with the most common being falls from height in younger children, sports-related injuries in adolescents and assault/motor vehicle

collisions in the later teenage years.[4] These fractures can occur in isolation but are also often a part of more complex facial fractures such as nasoorbitoethmoid fractures. The treatment of these injuries depends on the severity of the injury, degree of displacement, functional impairment, and age of the patient.

NASAL DEVELOPMENT/ANATOMY

The newborn pediatric nose is more protected from injury due to its lesser projection from the face, mainly cartilaginous structure, and increased prominence of the frontal bone/supraorbital rims due to the increased cranial/facial ratio in infants.[6] In young children, the paired nasal bones are also separated in the midline by a patent suture and much of the nasal septum is cartilaginous and unossified. Due to these anatomical differences, the nose is less likely to take the brunt of facial

a Division of Plastic Surgery, Department of Otolaryngology–Head and Neck Surgery, Seattle Childrens Hospital, Craniofacial Center; b Division of Plastic and Reconstructive Surgery, Department of Surgery, University of Washington; c Department of Otolaryngology–Head and Neck Surgery, University of Washington, Seattle Children's Hospital
* Corresponding author. Department of Otolaryngology–Head and Neck Surgery, University of Washington, Seattle Childrens Hospital, 1959 Northeast Pacific Street, Box 356515, Seattle, WA 98195.
E-mail address: Randall.bly@seattlechildrens.org

Oral Maxillofacial Surg Clin N Am 35 (2023) 577–584
https://doi.org/10.1016/j.coms.2023.04.005
1042-3699/23/© 2023 Elsevier Inc. All rights reserved.

impact and is more pliable to distribute forces and resist fracture. However, because there is a lack of ossified overlying nasal bone structure, much of this force is transmitted to the septum, which can result in increased injury or dislocation. This may go unnoticed at the time of the incident but can lead to significant growth and functional disturbance later in life.[7]

The nose then undergoes 2 distinct growth phases from 2 to 5 years of age and again during puberty reaching its adult size at approximately 16 to 18 years in girls and 18 to 20 years in boys.[8] Much of this growth has been purported to be from growth centers in the nasal septum located at the spheno-septal and septopremaxillary areas.[6,9] The latter area is also hypothesized to be integral in maxillary and overall midface growth.[9] Fractures to the pediatric nasal septum may result in potential growth disturbances and delayed deformities due to altered growth patterns.[10] It is challenging to know which is most impactful to growth—the initial trauma, the surgical repair, or the impact on airflow. Normal growth is likely multifactorial. In addition to an intact growth center, the ability to breathe more air through the nasal airway is likely a major contributor to normal growth and development. Restoring normal nasal airflow is a key factor in the decision for treatment in a young patient.

As children reach their teenage years, their nasal anatomy becomes more consistent with the adult nose. Externally, the upper third of the nose comprises paired nasal bones, the middle third with support from upper lateral cartilages, and lower third from lower lateral cartilages. The nasal septum has much more ossified bony support with the perpendicular plate of the ethmoid and vomer comprising the posterior septum and quadrangular cartilage making up the anterior portion. The nose is rich in blood supply with branches of the external and internal carotid contributing to its vascularity. The confluence of 5 terminal branches in the anterior septum (superior labial, anterior and posterior ethmoidal, greater palatine, and sphenopalatine) represents Kiesselbach's plexus, which is the source of most nasal bleeds (epistaxis).[11]

DIAGNOSIS

As with all trauma patients, the initial evaluation of the pediatric craniofacial trauma patient should follow Pediatric Advanced Life Support guidelines and include a primary and secondary survey ensuring intact airway, breathing, circulation, and evaluation of neurological status and any other concomitant injuries. Ensuring an adequate airway is of utmost importance because the pediatric airway is narrower and more collapsible.[12] In addition, infants are obligate nasal breathers and obstruction of the nasal airway due to trauma that otherwise could be tolerated in an adult can lead to severe feeding challenges, or even respiratory collapse in an infant.[12] After the patient has been stabilized, a focused history and physical of the head and neck can be performed. A thorough clinical history should be performed to understand the nature of the injury. Although it is rare for child abuse to be the cause of pediatric facial trauma, it should always be considered, and appropriate referrals placed if it is suspected.[13]

History

Questioning should highlight the mechanism of injury, timing, presence of nasal obstruction and whether any subjective change to the appearance of the nose has occurred. This can help elucidate the potential severity and/or morphology of potential underlying fractures to the nasal bridge or septum. Preinjury photographs can be extremely helpful to assess any changes from preinjury state and set expectations for posttreatment appearance.

The presence of epistaxis can be a particularly important finding. Although epistaxis can be present from soft tissue injury alone, it is almost always present in the setting of underlying nasal fracture/septal disruption, and as such, it is rare to have a fracture in the absence of nasal bleeding. Other findings such as vision changes, salty taste in the throat, and clear nasal drainage may help elucidate concomitant injuries such as orbital fractures, basilar skull fractures, cribriform plate fractures, or cerebrospinal fluid (CSF) leaks, respectively. If these are suspected, further imaging or diagnostic workup may be necessary.

The diagnosis of CSF leaks can be challenging to differentiate from normal clear mucous drainage. Some possible ancillary studies/findings include the "halo sign" from placing drainage on filter paper. Because CSF diffuses faster than blood or mucous, there should be a central area of blood surrounded by an outer ring of CSF. This however has shown to have poor sensitivity and specificity because water, saline, and other watery substances diffuse at a similar rate to CSF.[14] Some also advocate for testing the nasal drainage for glucose or beta-2-transferrin; however, the former has poor sensitivity/specificity and the latter although highly sensitive and specific is often not necessary, requires 1 mL of fluid, and can take up to a week to result.[15] Perhaps, the simplest approach is continued observation after cross-sectional imaging because nasal drainage will often abate after a few days, whereas CSF leak will usually be persistent/consistent.

Pain that is increasing after injury should raise suspicion for septal hematoma. Normally, after the trauma, there is gradually decreasing pain. If a patient returns with severe pain within the first few days after injury, a septal hematoma may be present.

Examination

As with any evaluation, a consistent and reproducible approach will allow for improved accuracy and prevent missing critical findings on examination. This should include evaluation of the entire head and neck to rule out any other injuries. It is common to focus on obvious deformity and miss important concomitant injuries. Specifically for suspected nasal fractures this can begin with inspection in the anteroposterior, sagittal and worms eye views assessing for edema, ecchymosis, evidence of previous epistaxis (dried blood at the nares), and obvious deviation of the nasal dorsum and septum. Depending on the timing of presentation, postinjury edema may obscure gross deformities. Moreover, due to the more pliable nature of nasal tissues in children the underlying cartilaginous septum may fracture/displace with no obvious external signs/symptoms.[8] A subtly displaced nasal dorsum may be suggestive of an underlying nasal septal dislocation/fracture but symptoms of septal deviation/obstruction may not become more apparent until the subsequent 2 to 3 days. An assessment of nasal airway patency is important, especially in infants. To do this, the child can be observed feeding, which is a time of obligatory nasal breathing. A helpful technique is to use a stethoscope that the tubing can be detached from the bell. Placing the end of the tubing directly to the nose allows the examiner to isolate the location and strength of audible airflow between left and right nares. Close follow-up for repeat evaluation and examination is therefore important.

Intranasal inspection should then be performed with a nasal speculum and proper lighting. Adequate pain control and often moderate sedation may be necessary to perform this depending on the child's age. Evaluation for septal deviation or nasal blockage may indicate a fractured septum. Persistent clear nasal drainage can be a sign of an underlying CSF leak or cribriform plate fracture and should be managed as above. Lacerations, bleeding, unilateral deviation of the septum, or focal swelling of the septal mucosa may indicate the presence of a septal hematoma. Although septal hematomas are a rare complication of nasal trauma, they have been shown to be more common in children.[8] Appropriate and timely diagnosis/treatment is quintessential to prevent septal necrosis, abscess, loss of septal support,

and late deformity such as collapse of the nasal dorsum or "saddle nose deformity."

Palpation of the nasal bones, septum, anterior nasal spine, and anterior tip of the nose evaluating for tenderness, step-offs, or mobility can also indicate an underlying fracture or septal pathologic condition. Palpation and inspection should then be continued throughout the remainder of the craniofacial skeleton because it is important to rule out concomitant injuries. Racoon eyes, battle sign, and hemotympanum may indicate a basilar skull fracture. Midface mobility or dental malocclusion may indicate concomitant maxillary fracture. A thorough eye examination including inspection for symmetry, visual acuity, extraocular eye movements, and pupillary examination should be performed on every child to rule out underlying orbital or ocular pathologic condition. Change in position of the orbits, telecanthus, or gaze restriction may indicate an underlying orbital fracture. Finally, a detailed neurologic examination assessing the 12 cranial nerves should also be evaluated.

In cases of suspected nasal bone fractures, imaging may not always be necessary but it is often obtained by the emergency department before consultation. Physical examination findings alone should be sufficient for diagnosis.[16] Plain films are of limited benefit because they have poor detail and in the setting of a primarily cartilaginous structure in children have a low sensitivity.[17] Some authors argue that ultrasound provides better detail than plain films, although its sensitivity is also low making it questionable in terms of clinical usefulness.[18] If there is a concern due to a higher energy mechanism of injury or signs of other concomitant injuries, a high-resolution computed tomography should be performed for a better evaluation of the underlying bony architecture and for better surgical and procedural planning.

TREATMENT
Epistaxis

Epistaxis, or nosebleed, can typically be controlled by applying direct pressure to both nasal alae for at least 10 minutes. For persistent nasal bleeding, the use of topical decongestants such as oxymetazoline, or anterior nasal packing may be helpful.[11] In severe cases, where an uncontrollable nasal bleed is occurring, it is essential to secure the airway and perform endoscopy to either isolate the source of bleeding or perform adequate packing, including a possible posterior nasal pack.

Septal Hematomas

Septal hematomas are more common in children than in adults due to the more cartilaginous nature of the septum causing buckling/underlying injury without disruption of the mucosa.[8] Septal hematomas must be promptly decompressed and managed quickly to prevent further complications. This can be done by draining the hematoma through a mucoperichondrial incision, followed by nasal packing or transseptal "through and through" quilting sutures to decrease the risk of recurrence.[19] The patient should be examined the next day after drainage to confirm that it has not reaccumulated. Children should be treated with antibiotics, such as augmentin, to prevent infection and septal abscess formation.[19] After the procedure, it is important to follow the child for 12 to 18 months to evaluate for any late deformities.[20] Early intervention and proper management of septal hematomas can help prevent long-term nasal deformities and maintain the normal structure and function of the nose (**Fig. 1**).

Observation/conservative management

After initial stabilization and repair of any acute injuries (lacerations, septal hematoma, epistaxis, and so forth) and diagnosis of nasal fracture is suspected, the next step is to determine whether intervention is necessary and if so, the optimal timing. If seen immediately after the injury evaluation of gross deformity, nasal obstruction or displacement may be feasible. Otherwise, swelling begins to distort/mask the deformity and nasal obstruction becomes nearly universal. This further stresses the importance of close follow up 3 to 5 days after swelling resolution for repeat evaluation. If no significant nasal deformity, nasal bone or septal deviation or functional impact to the nose is noted, further treatment may not be necessary. Infant nasoseptal deformities or fractures are rare and can often be observed if the infant is able to feed adequately.[21] Regardless, the patient should be informed to follow up in the future if they notice any deformity or functional limitations that develop as they age due to possible damage to the underlying growth centers as mentioned previously[6] (**Fig. 2**).

Closed reduction of nasal fractures

If significant displacement of the nasal bones or septum is present and functional symptoms persist, intervention should be pursued. The majority of nasoseptal fractures can and should be treated with closed reduction. This should be performed after 3 to 5 days to allow swelling to subside but before 7 to 10 days because children heal quickly and the fractured segments may become difficult to mobilize after that time.[6–8] Although closed reduction can be performed on an awake adult patient under local anesthesia, pediatric patients typically require general anesthesia.

The closed nasoseptal reduction technique involves several important steps. First, local anesthesia to the external nasal and infraorbital nerves and nasal packing with a vasoconstrictor, such as oxymetazoline, is administered for pain relief and improved visualization during the procedure. Bimanual pressure is applied to the nasal bones along with intranasal pressure using a Boies elevator (or other blunt nasal elevator) to apply right-left and anterior-posterior directed force to reduce the bones back into their preinjury position. Before attempting reduction, the elevator should be placed externally on the nose with the tip at the level of the medial canthus and the finger or tape placed at the nostril as a reference point to avoid damage to the skull base or cribriform plate from inserting the instrument too caudal. An Asch or Walsham forceps can then be used to grasp both sides of the septum and manipulate it into a straightened position in the midline as needed. It is important to note that if the underlying septal deformity is not corrected, the overlying nasal bones tend to fall back out of position.[22]

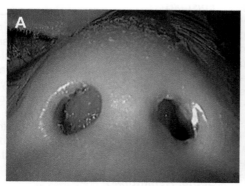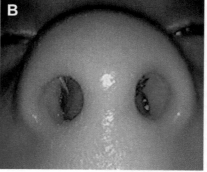

Fig. 1. A 3-year-old patient 2 weeks after nasal trauma developed an abscess where a nasal septal hematoma had occurred (*A*). She underwent operative drainage and silastic splints were placed to prevent reaccumulation in this endoscopic photograph (*B*). She healed well without nasal septal perforation.

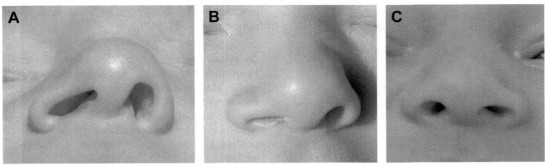

Fig. 2. Two photographs (*A*) and (*B*) of a 9-day old infant's nose with nasoseptal deformity that was present since vaginal delivery birth. She was born full-term and there was no reported birth trauma. She had mild stertor with breathing through nose while feeding. Nasal taping (cartilage molding) was discussed but ultimately the family elected for observation. A follow-up photograph just 11 days (*C*) later showed significant spontaneous improvement in nasal shape and symmetry, which continued to improve over time. The patient no longer has nasal airway symptoms.

After adequate repositioning of the nasal bones and septum, an external nasal splint should be placed with care taken to avoid medially displacing lateralized nasal bones from external pressure during application. If needed the blunt elevator can again be used to apply counterpressure intranasally during splint application. In cases where septal repositioning was performed, many authors advocate for the placement of silastic intranasal stents to help bolster the septal position during healing[7,8] (**Fig. 3**).

Acute/subacute limited open septorhinoplasty
The addition of this procedure to closed reduction of nasal fractures (CRNF) should be approached with caution due to the presence of growth centers in the nose that can be easily disrupted. Most surgeons advocate for delaying open septorhinoplasty until after puberty or closer to skeletal maturity to reduce the risk of injury.[6–8,10] However, there may be certain situations where limited septorhinoplasty is necessary, such as in cases of nonreducible anteroposterior septal displacement, severe nasal obstruction, chronic mouth breathing, or chronic refractory sinus disease.[7,8] In such cases, a limited septal approach such as a Killian/hemi-transfixion incision should be used to avoid the nasomaxillary junction growth center.[7,9] Use of the endoscope to improve visualization can minimize the amount of dissection

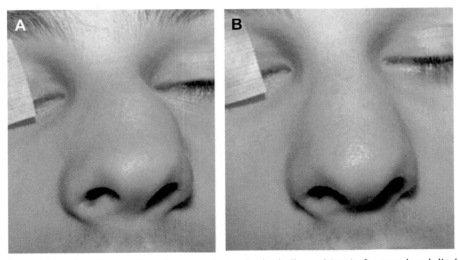

Fig. 3. A 16-year-old male patient suffered trauma during basketball, resulting in fractured and displaced nasal bones and fracture of nasal septum. He had symptoms of nasal obstruction in addition to the deformity shown in photograph (*A*). He underwent closed reduction of nasal and septal fractures in the operating room with adequate positioning of nasal bones and septum (*B*).

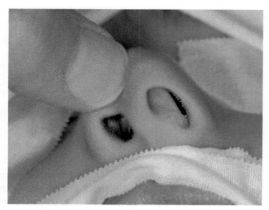

Fig. 4. A patient with severe septal deformity likely secondary to remote trauma. The caudal septum is completely deflected off the nasal spine. This required dissection of mucosa off the caudal septum and inserting it into a space created between the medial crura and suture in place to midline.

required and allow the operation to focus on the specific area of obstruction. Care should also be taken to preserve as much cartilage as possible with particular attention to the bony-cartilaginous junction, which is thought to be another growth center of the nose[6] (**Fig. 4**).

Delayed/late presenting open septorhinoplasty
Even after closed nasal reduction many patients continue to have or develop acquired nasal deformities and/or dysfunction as they grow. Although specific data for pediatric patients is limited, the literature suggests persistent nasal deformity/obstruction after closed reduction to be as high as 11% to 41%.[23–25] Due to this, septorhinoplasty at skeletal maturity is an especially important part of the treatment of these injuries. Parents should be informed of this possibility and encouraged to continue to monitor their child for new symptoms or deformity as they age.

Once completion of the pubertal growth phase has completed and patients near skeletal maturity, open septorhinoplasty can be considered. Many patients may present for the first time in adulthood with posttraumatic nasal deformity from an injury sustained during childhood. In either setting, formal open septorhinoplasty can be safely undertaken without fear of stunting underlying growth. The procedure can involve a range of functional and

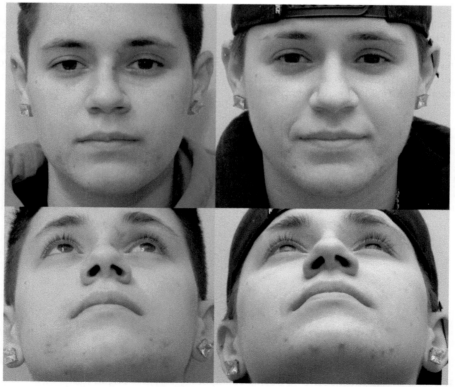

Fig. 5. A 23-year-old patient presenting with remote history of nasal trauma with C-shaped nasal dorsum deviation. Surgery involved an endonasal approach with lateral and medial osteotomies and septoplasty with left-sided endonasal spreader graft to aid in correcting asymmetric midvault collapse.

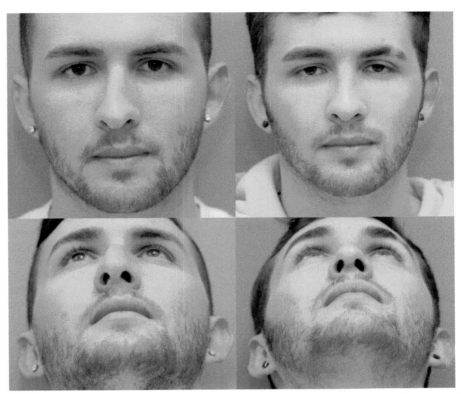

Fig. 6. A 27-year-old patient presenting with history of childhood trauma with sloping deviation of the nasal dorsum to the right. He underwent open approach with bilateral lateral and medial osteotomies, left-sided intermediate osteotomy given relative lengthening of the nasal bone on this side, caudal septal repositioning onto the maxillary spine, and bilateral extended spreader grafts to aid in correction of caudal septal deflection.

aesthetic techniques such as bony osteotomies for nasal bridge repositioning, submucous septal resection/repositioning, spreader grafts for opening of the internal nasal valve, and various cartilage grafts and suture techniques for alar, columellar, and tip refinement. A complete description of these techniques is beyond the scope of this article but should be considered as part of the overall surgical plan (**Figs. 5** and **6**).

SUMMARY

The evaluation and management of pediatric nasoseptal fractures requires a different approach compared with adult patients. Pediatric nasal fractures become increasingly more common after the first nasal/midface growth spurt around age 5 and make up nearly one-third of all pediatric facial fractures. The nasal septum is a crucial growth center for nasal and midface development, and any disturbance in potential growth must be considered when evaluating the injury and deciding on possible surgical manipulation. Prompt intervention is crucial to avoid late deformities, and imaging is not always necessary or helpful in diagnosis. It is important however to rule out any other concomitant injuries and obtain detailed imaging when higher severity injury is suspected. Closed reduction and splinting can treat most isolated pediatric nasoseptal fractures. However, open septorhinoplasty, performed after skeletal maturity, is an important aspect of treating pediatric nasal bone fractures because many patients may develop or have persistent nasal deformity and dysfunction even after closed reduction.

CLINICS CARE POINTS

- Nasal fracture makes up one third of all pediatric facial fractures.
- Septal hematoma requires prompt treatment to prevent negative sequalae.
- Restoring bilateral nasal airflow is likely an important component to normal nasal and facial growth.

DISCLOSURES

Dr R.A. Bly is cofounder and holds a financial interest of ownership equity with Wavely Diagnostics, Inc and EigenHealth, Inc. He is Consultant and stockholder, Spiway, LLC. All other authors report no disclosures.

FUNDING

Dr Bly was supported by the Washington Research Foundation, Seattle Children's Research Institute, Research Integration Hub.

REFERENCES

1. National Hospital Ambulatory Medical Care Survey (NHAMCS). Center for disease control and prevention. Atlanta, GA: National Center for Health Statistics; 1999.
2. Imahara SD, Hopper RA, Wang J, et al. Patterns and outcomes of pediatric facial fractures in the United States: a survey of the National Trauma Data Bank, J Am Coll Surg, 207 (5), 2008, 710–716.
3. Vyas RM, Dickinson BP, Wasson KL, et al. Pediatric facial fractures: current national incidence, distribution, and health care resource use, J Craniofac Surg, 19 (2), 2008, 339–349, [discussion: 350].
4. Cakabay T, Ustun Bezgin S. Pediatric nasal traumas: contribution of epidemiological features to detect the distinction between nasal fractures and nasal soft tissue injuries. J Craniofac Surg 2018;29(5): 1334–7.
5. Massenburg BB, Sanati-Mehrizy P, Taub PJ. Surgical treatment of pediatric craniofacial fractures: a national perspective. J Craniofac Surg 2015;26(8): 2375–80.
6. Verwoerd CD, Verwoerd-Verhoef HL. Rhinosurgery in children: basic concepts. Facial Plast Surg 2007;23(4):219–30.
7. Desrosiers AE 3rd, Thaller SR. Pediatric nasal fractures: evaluation and management. J Craniofac Surg 2011;22(4):1327–9.
8. Wright RJ, Murakami CS, Ambro BT. Pediatric nasal injuries and management. Facial Plast Surg 2011; 27(5):483–90.
9. Latham RA. Maxillary development and growth: the septopremaxillary ligament. J Anat 1970;107(Pt 3): 471–8.
10. Grymer LF, Gutierrez C, Stoksted P. Nasal fractures in children: influence on the development of the nose. J Laryngol Otol 1985;99:735–9.
11. Tabassom A. and Cho J.J., Epistaxis, In: Aboubakr S., StatPearls [internet], 2022, StatPearls Publishing; Treasure Island (FL), Available at: https://www.ncbi. nlm.nih.gov/books/NBK435997/.
12. Gassner R, Tuli T, Hächl O, et al. Craniomaxillofacial trauma in children: a review of 3,385 cases with 6,060 injuries in 10 years. J Oral Maxillofac Surg 2004;62(4):399.
13. Cole P, Kaufman Y, Hollier LH. Managing the pediatric facial fracture. Craniomaxillofacial Trauma Reconstr 2009;2(2):77–83.
14. Ray AM. Halo sign is neither sensitive nor specific for cerebrospinal fluid leak. Ann Emerg Med 2009; 53(2):288.
15. Chan DT, Poon WS, Ip CP, et al. How useful is glucose detection in diagnosing cerebrospinal fluid leak? The rational use of CT and Beta-2 transferrin assay in detection of cerebrospinal fluid fistula, Asian J Surg, 27 (1), 2004, 39–42.
16. Nigam A, Goni A, Benjamin A, et al. The value of radiographs in the management of the fractured nose. Arch Emerg Med 1993;10(4):293–7.
17. Stucker FJ Jr, Bryarly RC, Shockley WW. Management of nasal trauma in children. Arch Otolaryngol 1984;110(3):190–2.
18. Navaratnam R, Davis T. The role of ultrasound in the diagnosis of pediatric nasal fractures. J Craniofac Surg 2019;30(7):2099–101.
19. Sanyaolu LN, Farmer SE, Cuddihy PJ. Nasal septal haematoma. BMJ 2014;349:g6075.
20. Alvarez H, Osorio J, De Diego JI, et al. Sequelae after nasal septum injuries in children. Auris Nasus Larynx 2000;27(4):339–42.
21. Podoshin L, Gertner R, Fradis M, et al. Incidence and treatment of deviation of nasal septum in newborns. Ear Nose Throat J 1991;70(8):485–7.
22. Higuera S, Lee EI, Cole P, et al. Nasal trauma and the deviated nose, Plast Reconstr Surg, 120 (7 Suppl 2), 2007, 64S–75S.
23. Murray JA, Maran AG. The treatment of nasal injuries by manipulation. J Laryngol Otol 1980; 94(12):1405–10.
24. Kang BH, Kang HS, Han JJ, et al. A retrospective clinical investigation for the effectiveness of closed reduction on nasal bone fracture, Maxillofac Plast Reconstr Surg, 41 (1), 2019, 53.
25. Wang W, Lee T, Kohlert S, et al. Nasal fractures: the role of primary reduction and secondary revision. Facial Plast Surg 2019;35(6):590–601.

Pediatric Orbital Fractures

Bashar Hassan, MD[a,b], Fan Liang, MD[a,b], Michael P. Grant, MD, PhD, FACS[a,*]

KEYWORDS

- Pediatric orbital fractures • Orbital fractures in children • Pediatric orbital wall fractures
- Orbital wall fractures in children

KEY POINTS

- Different orbital wall fracture patterns exist in children, compared with adults, due to the unique anatomy and physiology of their developing craniofacial skeleton.
- A thorough history and physical examination are essential in the assessment of children with suspected orbital fractures.
- Physicians should be aware of symptoms and signs suggestive of trapdoor fractures with soft tissue entrapment that should prompt surgery within 48 hours of injury.
- Equivocal radiologic evidence of trapdoor fractures with soft tissue entrapment should not withhold surgery; imaging should only supplement the overall clinical picture.
- A multidisciplinary approach is recommended for the accurate diagnosis and proper management of pediatric orbital fractures.

BACKGROUND

Although the orbit is a commonly fractured region of the face in both the pediatric and adult populations, there are significant differences in the clinical presentation, management, and outcomes between these two patient populations. This is attributed, in part, to anatomical and physiological differences between the developing pediatric skeleton versus adult skull. Despite the advancements in craniomaxillofacial surgery in children, the choice of operative management of pediatric orbital fractures (POF), as well as surgical timing, remain areas of controversy and active research. Only a minority of pediatric patients present with absolute indications for reduction and internal fixation of POF, whereas the majority of patients present with a more complicated clinical picture. Workup of POF can be further complicated by limitations in patient compliance to physical examination and imaging, leading to missed diagnoses. In POF, the decision to operate must balance surgical and anesthetic risk with potential benefits of intervention, such as the prevention of ocular motility disorders and globe malposition. In this article, we highlight the unique aspects of POF with regard to epidemiology, anatomy, clinical presentation, assessment, surgical indications, and complications.

EPIDEMIOLOGY

According to a review of the National Trauma Data Bank based on 12,739 pediatric patients with facial fractures, POF was the least common fracture type (9%) compared with mandibular (32.7%), nasal (30.2%), and maxillary/zygomatic (28.6%) pediatric facial fractures (**Fig. 1**).[1] In other studies, POF ranged from 5% to 56% of pediatric facial fractures.[2–4] The incidence of POF varies according to age, sex, etiology, season of the year, and fracture site. Although several attempts have been made to quantify the characteristics and outcomes surrounding POF, the topic on a whole is significantly less well researched than adult orbital fractures; evidence on POF and its relation to the aforementioned factors is based on either small case series investigating POF or large trauma series investigating pediatric facial fractures in general.

[a] Division of Plastic and Reconstructive Surgery, R Adams Cowley Shock Trauma Center, University of Maryland Medical Center, 110 South Paca Street, Baltimore, MD, USA; [b] Department of Plastic and Reconstructive Surgery, Johns Hopkins Hospital, 600 North Wolfe Street, Baltimore, MD, USA
* Corresponding author. 110 South Paca Street, Suite 4-S-124, Baltimore, MD, 21201.
E-mail address: michael.grant@som.umaryland.edu

Oral Maxillofacial Surg Clin N Am 35 (2023) 585–596
https://doi.org/10.1016/j.coms.2023.05.002
1042-3699/23/© 2023 Elsevier Inc. All rights reserved.

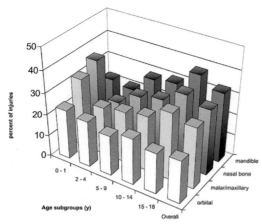

percent of injuries

Age subgroups (y)

0 - 1
2 - 4
5 - 9
10 - 14
15 - 18
Overall

mandible
nasal bone
malar/maxillary
orbital

Fig. 1. The incidence of pediatric orbital fractures (%) stratified by fracture site and age (years). (*From* Imahara SD, Hopper RA, Wang J, Rivara FP, Klein MB. Patterns and outcomes of pediatric facial fractures in the United States: a survey of the National Trauma Data Bank [published correction appears in J Am Coll Surg.2009 Feb;208(2):325]. J Am Coll Surg. 2008;207(5):710-716.)

In general, POF is often more likely to occur in boys[3,5–10] and during the summertime.[11] The most common etiology of POF has been attributed to activities of daily living,[7] assault,[5,12,13] sports injuries,[14] falls,[15] or motor vehicle collision.[6,8,16] This inconsistency regarding the most common etiology of POF might be due to the different age groups analyzed by the different studies, because the etiology of pediatric facial fracture has been shown to vary according to the child's age.[17]

Facial fractures, including orbital fractures, are significantly less common in children compared with adults.[3,18,19] Only 1% of facial fractures have been reported to occur in children aged younger than 1 year.[20] Although the overall incidence of POF does not seem to significantly vary across age groups in children (see **Fig. 1**), different age groups tend to have different POF patterns. For example, orbital roof fractures are predominant in children aged younger than 7 to 10 years compared with orbital floor fractures, which become more common afterwards and with increasing age.[3,7,8,13–15,21] This is attributed to the changing anatomy and physiology of the developing craniofacial skeleton which will be discussed below.

DEVELOPMENT AND ANATOMY
The Neurocranium and Face

The human skull is composed of the neurocranium and the facial skeleton. Neurocranial development is continuous, driven by the enlarging brain, and occurs in all directions. The majority of neurocranial development occurs before the age of 2 years, at which the neurocranium reaches around 75% of its adult size. Neurocranial growth then gradually decreases and is 95% complete by the age of 10. The facial skeleton, in contrast, has discontinuous growth and shows vectored expansion along various anatomic sites. It is driven by bone apposition, resorption, and affected by hormonal changes during puberty. The majority of facial skeletal development occurs before the age of 5 years, at which the facial skeleton reaches around 80% of its adult size.[22,23] Facial skeletal development decreases thereafter before accelerating again at puberty and abates around the age of 17 years. The asynchronous growth of the neurocranium and facial skeletons results in various neurocranium-to-face size ratios of 8-to-1 at birth, 4-to-1 at the age of 5 years, and 2.5-to-1 in adulthood (**Fig. 2**A, B, D, respectively).[8,22,24] This difference in neurocranium-to-face size ratios is one reason behind the greater incidence of intracranial injury and craniofacial to maxillofacial fractures in children compared with adults.[3,18,19,25,26]

Another reason for the difference in susceptibility to facial fractures, including orbital fractures, is the differences in facial bone composition and resultant changes in mechanical properties in children compared with adults.[9] The process of bone mineralization, which mainly occurs after 2 to 3 years of age, transforms the immature, elastic, and cancellous bone of the growing facial skeleton into the mature, mineralized, and cortical bone of the adult facial skeleton.[8,27] This provides the pediatric facial bones with a greater ability to bend, rather than break, and withstand traumatic forces compared with adult facial bones. As a result, children are more likely to develop incomplete fractures, also known as "greenstick" fractures, compared with adults.[16] The bony composition of the pediatric facial skeleton also confers the advantage of greater bone healing and remodeling, which supports the nonoperative management of pediatric facial fractures. However, the elasticity of the pediatric facial skeleton, as well as the presence of rudimentary sinuses, permits an easier transmission of traumatic forces to the neurocranium increasing the risk of intracranial injury.[7]

The Orbit and Adjacent Sinuses

The 2 orbits are a pair of quadrangular truncated pyramids whose contents are arranged according to the rule of 7; there are 7 bones, 7 intraorbital muscles, and 7 nerves in the orbit.[28] The 7 bones of the orbit are the frontal, maxillary, zygomatic,

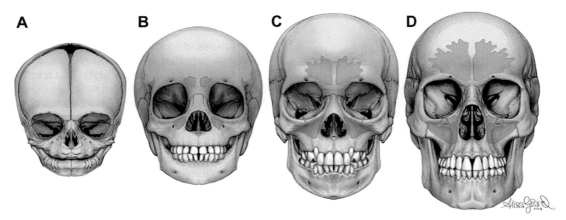

Fig. 2. Craniofacial development. Cranium to face ratio at birth (*A*) is 8:1 and evolves to 2.5:1 at adulthood (*D*). Maxillary sinus (blue) progressive pneumatization at birth (*A*), 5 years of age (*B*), 12 years of age (*C*), and adulthood (*D*). Frontal sinus (pink) progressive pneumatization at 5 years of age (*B*), 12 years of age (*C*), and adulthood (*D*). (Illustration courtesy of Alisa O. Girard, MD.)

ethmoid, lacrimal, palatine, and greater and lesser wings of the sphenoid. These bones make up the 4 orbital walls (roof, floor, lateral wall, and medial wall) and the first 3 make up the outer orbital rim.

As the facial skeleton develops, paranasal sinuses undergo pneumatization, and the orbital walls change configuration and thickness. Three of the 4 orbital walls (roof, floor, and medial wall) are adjacent to paranasal sinuses (**Fig. 3**). Initially, the sinuses and the nasal cavity are merged in utero, until the frontal, maxillary, and ethmoid sinuses separate from the nasal cavity in the second trimester. The maxillary sinuses are the first to pneumatize and expand rapidly from birth to 3 years of age and from 7 to 12 years of age. The intermediary delay in maxillary sinus pneumatization coincides with a period of mixed dentition where the unerupted maxillary teeth are immediately below the orbital floor, shielding it and mitigating fracture risk. The subsequent resumption of maxillary sinus pneumatization beyond 7 years coincides with eruption of permanent dentition and ends at 16 to 18 years of age when it reaches adult size. In contrast to the biphasic growth pattern of the maxillary sinuses, the ethmoid sinuses continuously expand from birth to 12 years of age. As the ethmoid sinuses pneumatize, the medial orbital walls gradually become thinner and more susceptible to fracture (see **Fig. 3**). The maxillary and ethmoid sinuses growth patterns thus help explain the greater susceptibility of children aged older than 10 to 12 years to orbital floor and medial wall fractures.[3,8,13,14,21,29]

The frontal sinuses start to pneumatize around 5 to 7 years of age (see **Fig. 2**B).[30] Before that, the lack of well-developed frontal sinuses allows facial traumatic forces to be directly transmitted to the orbital roof without force dissipation. This phenomenon, as well as the high cranium-to-face ratio discussed earlier, explains the greater susceptibility of children aged younger than 7 years to orbital roof fractures, as previously mentioned.[7,8,15]

The orbital cavity contains the globe, vessels, nerves, extraocular muscles, tendons, lacrimal gland, trochlea, periorbital fat, and other connective tissues. The orbital septum, check ligaments, and Lockwood's suspensory ligament constitute the periorbital structures that provide ligamentous support to the globe. These periorbital soft tissues retain elasticity that helps provide stability, resist traumatic forces, protect the pediatric orbit against fractures, and even splint orbital contents in case of fractures (**Fig. 4**). This characteristic of periorbital soft tissues may explain the relatively lower incidence of enophthalmos in children. Besides the bone composition of the pediatric facial skeleton discussed earlier, the resilience of the periorbital soft tissue also supports the nonoperative management of pediatric facial and orbital fractures.

PRESENTATION AND ASSESSMENT

The presentation of pediatric orbital and facial fractures is significantly different than that of adult orbital and facial fractures due to the previously discussed differences in the anatomy and physiology of the growing facial skeleton. The elasticity of the pediatric facial skeleton makes it less prone to fractures compared with the adult facial skeleton. Therefore, when pediatric facial fractures occur, strong traumatic forces are usually the cause and associated injuries should be suspected. It was reported that among children presenting with POF,

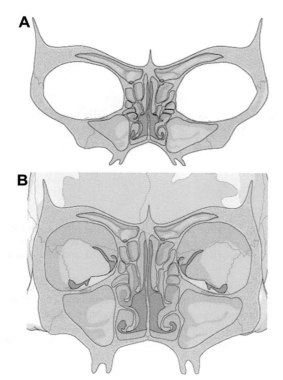

Fig. 3. The evolution of the orbital walls and sinuses and differences between children and adults. The orbital floor becomes deeper and its most inferior point shifts posteriorly. The orbital medial wall becomes thinner, whereas the orbital roof becomes thicker in adults. (*From* Oppenheimer AJ, Monson LA, Buchman SR. Pediatric orbital fractures. *Craniomaxillofac Trauma Reconstr.* 2013;6(1):9-20.)

43.4% had concomitant intracranial injury and 20% had significant injury beyond the head and neck. POF with concomitant head and/or chest injuries are significantly associated with greater odds of mortality.[7] Furthermore, a greater risk of concurrent intracranial injury is seen in patients presenting with fractures of multiple orbital walls.[6] Sobol and colleagues reported an interesting case of a 3-year-old child with combined orbital roof and floor fractures with concomitant epidural hemorrhage (**Fig. 5**).[31] When one orbital wall is fractured, practitioners should carefully assess the other orbital walls for concomitant fractures. Coon and colleagues found that around 40% of children presenting with orbital roof fractures also have another orbital wall fracture.[32] It is recognized that looking for associated fractures and injuries is challenging due to the generally uncooperative nature of pediatric patients. Nonetheless, a thorough traumatic survey and having a low threshold for obtaining radiographic imaging when facial fracture or intracranial injury is suspected are of paramount importance.

Orbital Floor Fractures

Orbital floor fractures can be classified as unentrapped/communited, also known as "open-door" fractures (see **Fig. 4**), or entrapped, known as "trapdoor" fractures (**Fig. 6**). The elastic nature of the growing facial skeleton predisposes to minimally displaced greenstick fractures compared with blowout fractures in adults. Greenstick fractures can recoil back to their initial position, *trapping* the bulging periorbital soft tissues, hence the *trapdoor* nomenclature and the preponderance of these fractures in the pediatric population.[5,13,33,34] The inferior rectus muscle depresses and adducts the eye. Patients with entrapped inferior rectus muscle often present with vertical gaze diplopia and restriction of upgaze/supraduction (see **Fig. 6**). This entrapment inflicts high compartment pressure on the

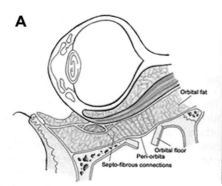
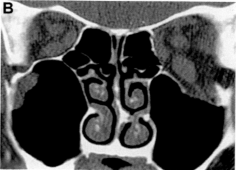

Fig. 4. (*A*) Pediatric open-door fracture with preservation of ligamentous support. Note the resilient periorbital soft tissue, which splints the orbital structures and globe in case of fractures. (*B*) Coronal CT image showing an equivalent orbital floor open-door fracture without muscle entrapment. ([*A*] *From* Losee JE, Afifi A, Jiang S, et al. Pediatric orbital fractures: classification, management, and early follow-up. Plast Reconstr Surg. 2008;122(3):886-897. (see **Fig. 4**A).)

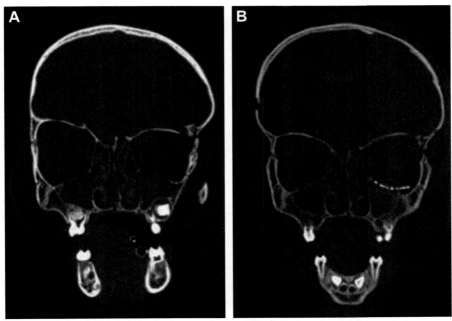

Fig. 5. (*A*) Coronal CT image demonstrating a displaced orbital roof blow-in fracture and large orbital floor blowout fracture preoperatively. (*B*) Coronal CT image following operative repair. (*From* Sobol DL, Lee A, Susarla SM. Unusual Combined Orbital Roof and Orbital Floor Fractures in A Pediatric Patient. Plast Reconstr Surg Glob Open. 2020;8(12):e3324. Published 2020 Dec 21.)

inferior rectus muscle and other periorbital soft tissues, potentially leading to ischemia and/or infarction and long-term motility problems. This is the reason extraocular muscle entrapment is considered a surgical emergency and should be addressed urgently. When blow-out fractures occur in pediatric patients (without extraocular muscle entrapment), enophthalmos and/or hypoglobus are rarely seen as presenting signs, due to the periorbital supporting structures described earlier that mitigate risk of globe malposition.

Patients with POF can present with classical symptoms and signs including pain, diplopia, limited extraocular motility, conjunctival erythema, subconjunctival hemorrhage, and periorbital soft tissue swelling. However, trapdoor fractures can cause entrapment and significant extraocular motility restriction without any periorbital ecchymosis, edema, conjunctival or subconjunctival abnormalities, or significant imaging findings. These trapdoor fractures are termed white-eyed fractures (see **Fig. 6**).[35] When muscle gets entrapped in trapdoor fractures, it may be engulfed with fat in between the muscle and bone. This makes it hard for the muscle to be visualized on traditional computed tomography (CT) scans, which is often missed in 50% of the cases of muscle entrapment.[36] One study revealed that patients with white-eyed fractures were less likely to undergo orbital imaging in the emergency department, less likely to be seen urgently by an ophthalmologist, and had a 4 to 5 days delay in follow-up with

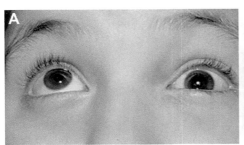
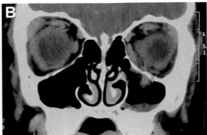

Fig. 6. (*A*) Child with "white-eyed" left orbital trapdoor fracture with loss of left supraduction. Note the lack of conjunctival erythema, subconjunctival hemorrhage, and periorbital edema. (*B*) Coronal CT image showing entrapment of the left inferior rectus muscle under a small left orbital floor fracture.

an ophthalmologist compared with other patients.[37] Hence, practitioners should not solely rely on overt ocular abnormalities, like subconjunctival hemorrhage, or radiographic evidence alone for the diagnosis of entrapment. Instead, a thorough physical examination with a proper assessment of extraocular muscle motility should be performed and supplemented with radiographic evidence to arrive at an accurate diagnosis and management plan.[36] Surgery within 24 to 48 hours of presentation for patients presenting with white-eyed fractures is favorable and leads to better long-term motility compared with surgery after 2 weeks of presentation.[35]

Another potential manifestation of trapdoor fractures is the oculocardiac reflex, characterized by the triad of bradycardia, nausea/vomiting, and syncope.[38] The extraocular muscle entrapment triggers an afferent signal via the ophthalmic division of the trigeminal nerve to the main sensory nucleus of the trigeminal nerve, which in turn sends back an efferent signal via the motor nucleus of the vagus nerve increasing parasympathetic tone and bradycardia. Of children with trapdoor fractures, it has been reported that 95% to 100% present with restricted extraocular motility[5,13] and that up to 63% present with nausea/vomiting.[5] Nausea/vomiting has been reported to have a positive predictive value of 83.3% for entrapment in trapdoor fractures.[38] Hence, the oculocardiac reflex has been considered as highly suggestive of inferior rectus entrapment and another indication for urgent surgical repair of POF.[39] Surgical intervention allows for the prompt resolution of the symptoms of the oculocardiac reflex.[13] This, again, signifies the importance of a thorough physical examination including assessment of vital signs, extraocular motility, visual acuity, forced ductions, and pupillary function for the diagnosis of possible extraocular muscle entrapment.

Orbital Medial Wall Fractures

Orbital medial wall fractures are prone to the entrapment of the medial rectus muscle (**Fig. 7**). The function of the medial rectus muscle is to adduct the eye. Patients with entrapped medial rectus muscle often present with horizontal diplopia and lateral gaze restriction (see **Fig. 7**A).

It is worth noting that the presentation of patients with medial rectus muscle entrapment differs depending on the type of medial rectus entrapment in the orbital medial wall fracture. An anterior entrapment of the taut medial rectus muscle results in restricted abduction. However, an entrapment with slack of the medial rectus muscle results in restricted adduction with no limitation to abduction, as is the case in **Fig. 7**.

Orbital Roof Fractures

As discussed earlier, the delay in frontal sinus pneumatization and the high cranium-to-face ratio in children aged younger than 7 years increase their risk of orbital roof fractures and concomitant intracranial injuries.

The most common fracture pattern involving the orbital roof in children extends along the frontal bone through the supraorbital foramen.[16] The superior oblique muscle, originating in the upper medial side of the orbit, abducts, depresses, and internally rotates the eye. Orbital roof fractures may be complicated by the entrapment of the superior oblique tendon causing restriction in supraduction during adduction, or what is known as "Brown syndrome" (**Fig. 8**).

Another manifestation of orbital roof fractures in children is the "blow-in" fracture. This is due to a supraorbital force directed inferiorly and causing the collapse of the orbital roof into the orbit. Children often present with periorbital edema and ecchymosis, upper eyelid pseudoptosis, restriction of upgaze/supraduction, dystopia, and

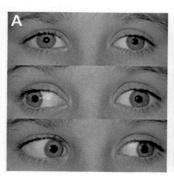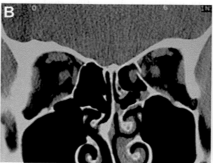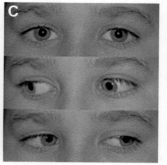

Fig. 7. (A) Child with left orbital medial wall fracture with loss of left adduction on right gaze (middle image). (B) Coronal CT image showing entrapment of the left medial rectus muscle with left orbital medial wall fracture. (C) Same child with restoration of motility after surgery.

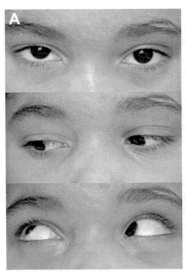
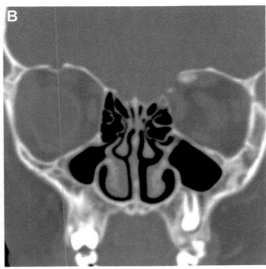

Fig. 8. (*A*) Child with left orbital roof fracture with restriction of left upgaze/supraduction on right gaze/adduction (bottom image). (*B*) Coronal CT image showing entrapment of the left superior oblique muscle with left orbital roof fracture.

diplopia (**Fig. 9**). Surgical repair is often indicated due to the compression of the orbital contents by the orbital roof fragments.

Imaging

High-resolution head CT scan has been considered the gold standard modality for radiographic evaluation of POF. Noncontrast CT has been shown to be highly sensitive (96%) and specific (71%) for the diagnosis of orbital floor fractures in adults.[40] However, the limitations of the use of noncontrast CT in the pediatric population include increased exposure of the developing lens to radiation, suboptimal visualization of soft tissues, and long scanning times. Alternatively, helical orbital CT scans with shorter scanning times and less motion artifact can be used.[41] As mentioned earlier, extraocular muscle and soft tissue entrapment may be underestimated on CT scans,[36] so high-resolution MRI combined with a microscopy orbital coil can be used as an alternative for better soft tissue depiction and less radiation exposure.[42] Although MRI and CT have similar sensitivities for

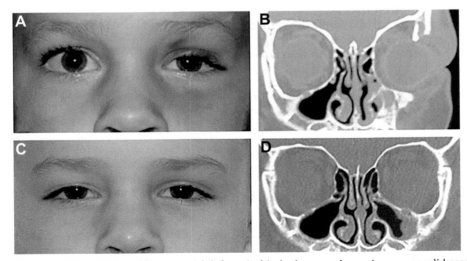

Fig. 9. (*A*) Child with left orbital roof fracture with left periorbital edema, ecchymosis, upper eyelid pseudoptosis, and dystopia. (*B*) Coronal CT image showing left orbital roof collapse. Note the orbital roof fragments causing downward compression of the orbital contents and globe leading to dystopia. (*C*) Same child with restoration of motility after surgery. (*D*) Coronal CT image showing restoration of orbital roof and globe position.

the detection of orbital floor fractures, CT has been shown to be superior in demonstrating small orbital and associated fractures and is relatively cheaper.[43] Even with the advancement of other imaging modalities, such as ultrasound, CT remains the imaging modality of choice for the detection of orbital fractures.[44] MRI can then supplement CT if soft tissue entrapment is suspected but not visualized.[43]

SURGICAL INDICATIONS

Surgeons managing POF have to weigh the postoperative complications of surgery versus surgical benefits and avoidance of long-term complications of late or no repair. Controversy still exists regarding the optimal timing of surgical intervention in the management of POF. However, most surgeons recommend urgent surgery, within 24 to 48 hours of presentation, in case of trapdoor fractures with extraocular muscle entrapment.[45–47] Studies have shown that surgery performed within 24 hours,[47] 2 to 4 days,[35] 7 days,[13] 8 days,[48] 14 days,[5,49] or 30 days,[49] of trapdoor fractures with periorbital tissue entrapment was associated with improved functional motility outcomes compared with surgery performed later. Late intervention increases the risk of ischemia, fibrosis, and callus formation at the fracture site, especially due to the fast turnover of the growing pediatric facial skeleton, which increases long-term complications and makes orbital fracture repair challenging.[33,50]

Hence, urgent surgery within 48 hours of periocular trauma is recommended if at least one of the following is present.

- Symptomatic diplopia with positive forced ductions on physical examination,[13,33,34,47,49,51]
- Confirmed periorbital soft tissue entrapment on imaging,
- Restricted ocular motility (regardless of conjunctival abnormalities) on physical examination with/without confirmed trapdoor fracture or soft tissue entrapment on imaging,[5,33–35,49,51–53]
- Oculocardiac reflex symptoms and/or signs with/without confirmed trapdoor fracture or soft tissue entrapment on imaging,[5,52]
- Acute vertical orbital dystopia, enophthalmos, or hypoglobus,[51,52] and
- Large orbital floor fractures—*due to concern for latent enophthalmos or hypoglobus.*[34,51,54]

The last surgical indication in this list is still controversial. In adults, operative management is recommended for orbital fractures greater than 2 to 3 cm^2 or involving 50% or more of the orbital wall.[55,56] However, the pediatric facial skeleton might impose different indications. Losee and colleagues and Kim and colleagues showed no significant difference in the incidence of enophthalmos with or without operative management of POF, regardless of the size of orbital floor fracture.[7,57] This is in contrast to 2 more recent studies by Broyles and colleagues and Coon and colleagues who showed significantly greater odds of globe malposition with nonoperative management of large orbital floor fractures.[51,54] We recommend early surgical intervention for restoration of the orbital anatomy to avoid soft tissue fibrosis and long-term complications in case of large orbital floor fractures. More evidence and larger studies are needed to determine if risk of globe malposition varies with orbital floor fracture size and the critical defect size for operative management.

Conversely, patients without diplopia or restricted ocular motility and radiographically nondisplaced or minimally displaced orbital fractures without evidence of extraocular muscle entrapment may be safely monitored for improvement without the need for urgent operative management.[5,7,52]

SURGICAL TECHNIQUE

Similar surgical techniques for the repair of orbital fractures are done in both children and adults. Different approaches (transconjunctival, transcaruncular, transcutaneous, or transantral) are required depending on the different orbital walls involved. The transconjunctival dissection is done through a posterior lamella incision in the preseptal or retroseptal plane. The transcutaneous dissection, however, is done through an anterior lamella incision. Surgical repair is usually done through a transconjunctival approach with or without lateral canthotomy/cantholysis for orbital floor fractures and through a transcaruncular approach for medial wall fractures. These approaches provide excellent direct visualization of the fracture. The transantral approach can also be used for posterior orbital floor repair but is rarely used by surgeons. The transcutaneous approach is rarely used too due to a greater risk of ectropion and eyelid retraction compared with other surgical approaches.

For orbital roof fracture repair, the passageway to the superolateral orbital rim leads from the skin incision through the orbicularis oculi muscle layer. Skin muscle flaps are raised leaving the orbital septum intact. The preaponeurotic space and the fat pads inside are not entered and serve as a buffer for critical underlying structures such as the levator aponeurosis. Gentle upward and lateral (temporal) traction of the wound edges facilitate access to the supraperiosteal plane over the lateral bony rim rapidly.

After exposure of the fracture, an implant should be placed, and the choice is dictated by the size and shape of the fracture. Several alloplastic (porous polyethylene, polyester urethane, titanium mesh, Supramid, GORE-TEX, Teflon, or silicone sheet) and autogenous (fascia lata, nasal septum, or iliac crest bone) materials can be used for repair of large POF. Small greenstick fractures, however, often do not require implant placement.[58] Alloplastic implants have several advantages over autogenous implants including greater durability, availability, tensile strength, and the option to choose between absorbable and nonabsorbable implants. Nonetheless, alloplastic implants carry an increased risk of extrusion, displacement, infection, and fibrosis.[58] Several studies have compared the different types of implants used for orbital fracture repair in adults[59–61]; however, much fewer studies investigated the outcomes following repair using different implants in the pediatric population. Abumanhal and colleagues reviewed children who had repair of orbital trapdoor fracture using the polyester urethane implant. After a median follow-up of 13.6 months, they reported residual diplopia in 3 patients but no enophthalmos or other postoperative complications associated with the material used.[62] The use of resorbable plates and screws for POF reconstruction has also been described but is not common in clinical practice due to concerns for globe malposition.[63,64]

ACUTE COMPLICATIONS

Acute complications following POF repair can either be iatrogenic or due to the initial traumatic injury. Among these complications, persistent diplopia is the most commonly reported postoperative complication, primarily due to trapdoor fractures with extraocular muscle ischemia/fibrosis due to a delayed repair and/or missed diagnosis.[58,65] This is particularly the case in children due to aforementioned reasons including the pediatric facial skeleton bone composition and regeneration. Treatment of persistent diplopia can be considered 6 months after surgery and involves specialized glasses and/or rebalancing extraocular muscles. Other acute complications include globe injury and/or malposition, optic nerve injury leading to vision loss, periorbital soft tissue injury, infraorbital dysesthesia, implant migration/extrusion, infection, orbital hemorrhage, and others.

POF may be associated with injury to the globe, including globe rupture, retinal, optic nerve, and ocular vessels. This indicates the importance of timely evaluation of patients presenting with POF by an ophthalmologist. The correction of neuro-visual disorders takes precedence over fracture reconstruction to decrease the risk of visual loss.

Iatrogenic complications are possible due to improper surgical technique or intraoperative injury to orbital structures. For example, a subciliary incision leads to a higher risk of cicatricial lower eyelid retraction, so the transconjunctival incision is preferred.[66,67] Postoperative diplopia and/or enophthalmos can also occur due to failure of proper bone defect coverage after replacing herniated orbital tissue during surgery. New onset unilateral vision loss can occur following orbital fracture repair due to increased pressure at the orbital apex, termed "orbital apex syndrome."[68] The most common cause of postoperative orbital apex syndrome is retrobulbar hemorrhage. Aside from acute vision loss, retrobulbar hemorrhage may be suspected due to sudden proptosis and/or periorbital ecchymosis and should prompt urgent lateral canthotomy/cantholysis for surgical decompression, and possibly optic nerve decompression.[69] Although this phenomenon is rare, it shows that postoperative clinical examination is as important as preoperative clinical examination in patients treated for orbital fractures and should always be performed.

LONG-TERM COMPLICATIONS

Late enophthalmos and/or hypoglobus are possible complications of large (>50% involvement) orbital wall fractures if not repaired early.[51,54] Several studies, however, did not find fracture size to be related to the development of late enophthalmos.[7,57,70] Delayed orbital tissue atrophy due to soft tissue injury was found to be the main predictor of late enophthalmos by Kim and colleagues. Because soft tissue atrophy is not preventable even with adequate soft tissue restoration and orbital bone reconstruction, Kim and colleagues recommend orbital overcorrection if there is evidence of soft tissue incarceration due to the risk of late enophthalmos despite orbital fracture repair.[57]

Iatrogenic long-term complications of orbital fracture repair include persistent ectropion (more common with transcutaneous incisions,[71] especially subciliary incisions),[72,73] entropion (more common with transconjunctival incisions), and hypertrophic scarring (more common with subtarsal incisions).[73] Canthopexy/canthoplasty can be performed for lower lids with significant laxity or weak tone to mitigate lower lid malposition. Early postoperative lower lid malposition can be addressed with conservative scar massage. Persistent postoperative lower lid malposition, however, may require anterior lamellar scar release with full-thickness skin grafting and/or lower lid tightening with canthopexy/canthoplasty.

As discussed previously, the use of alloplastic versus autogenous implants for POF reconstruction is associated with greater risk of extrusion, displacement, infection, and fibrosis. Autogenous implants have been the gold standard material for POF reconstruction due to better integration into surrounding bone, revascularization, and decreased risk of fibrosis.[74] Resorbable materials for POF reconstruction have been associated with globe malposition at 2 months because the plate dissolves and the tensile strength is lost, and local inflammatory reaction at 7 months.[63,64]

SUMMARY

POF can be challenging to diagnose and treat. Orbital fracture treatment algorithms in adults do not apply to children due to the different anatomy and physiology of the growing facial skeleton. A thorough history and physical examination are of paramount importance and can hint toward the presence of an orbital fracture with/without soft tissue entrapment. Symptomatic diplopia with positive forced ductions, restricted ocular motility (regardless of conjunctival abnormalities), nausea/vomiting, bradycardia, vertical orbital dystopia, enophthalmos, or hypoglobus are highly suggestive of a trapdoor fracture with soft tissue entrapment and should prompt surgery within 48 hours of injury. Evidence of trapdoor fracture with soft tissue entrapment on imaging is another surgical indication but equivocal results should not withhold surgery. Imaging should supplement the overall clinical picture and should not be solely relied on for the diagnosis of soft tissue entrapment. A multidisciplinary approach is recommended for the accurate diagnosis and proper management of POF.

CLINICS CARE POINTS

- When evaluating children with facial traumatic injury, look for symptoms/signs of trapdoor fractures with soft tissue entrapment: symptomatic diplopia with positive forced ductions, restricted ocular motility (regardless of conjunctival abnormalities), nausea/vomiting, bradycardia, vertical orbital dystopia, enophthalmos, and hypoglobus.
- Periorbital ecchymosis, edema, conjunctival/subconjunctival abnormalities, and significant imaging findings are not necessary for the diagnosis of trapdoor fractures with soft tissue entrapment in children.

- Do not withhold surgical intervention in children with suspected trapdoor fractures and soft tissue entrapment if radiologic evidence is absent/equivocal.
- Treat children with trapdoor fractures and soft tissue entrapment within 48 hours of injury.

DISCLOSURE

The authors have nothing to disclose.

ACKNOWLEDGMENTS

The authors would like to acknowledge the efforts of the medical illustrator of **Fig. 2**: Alisa Girard, MBS, Department of Plastic and Reconstructive Surgery, Johns Hopkins School of Medicine, Baltimore, Maryland, USA.

REFERENCES

1. Imahara SD, Hopper RA, Wang J, et al. Patterns and outcomes of pediatric facial fractures in the United States: a survey of the National Trauma Data Bank. J Am Coll Surg 2008;207(5):710–6. Epub 2008 Aug 9. Erratum in: J Am Coll Surg.2009;208(2):325.
2. Bales CR, Randall P, Lehr HB. Fractures of the facial bones in children. J Trauma 1972;12(1):56–66.
3. Posnick JC, Wells M, Pron GE. Pediatric facial fractures: evolving patterns of treatment. J Oral Maxillofac Surg 1993;51(8):836–44 [discussion: 844-5].
4. Grunwaldt L, Smith DM, Zuckerbraun NS, et al. Pediatric facial fractures: demographics, injury patterns, and associated injuries in 772 consecutive patients. Plast Reconstr Surg 2011;128(6):1263–71.
5. Bansagi ZC, Meyer DR. Internal orbital fractures in the pediatric age group: characterization and management. Ophthalmology 2000;107(5):829–36.
6. Donahue DJ, Smith K, Church E, et al. Intracranial neurological injuries associated with orbital fracture. Pediatr Neurosurg 1997;26(5):261–8.
7. Losee JE, Afifi A, Jiang S, et al. Pediatric orbital fractures: classification, management, and early follow-up. Plast Reconstr Surg 2008;122(3):886–97.
8. Koltai PJ, Amjad I, Meyer D, et al. Orbital fractures in children. Arch Otolaryngol Head Neck Surg 1995;121(12):1375–9.
9. McGraw BL, Cole RR. Pediatric maxillofacial trauma. Age-related variations in injury. Arch Otolaryngol Head Neck Surg 1990;116(1):41–5.
10. Baek SH, Lee EY. Clinical analysis of internal orbital fractures in children. Korean J Ophthalmol 2003;17(1):44–9.
11. Oppenheimer AJ, Monson LA, Buchman SR. Pediatric orbital fractures. Craniomaxillofac Trauma Reconstr

2013;6(1):9–20. https://doi.org/10.1055/s-0032-133 2213.

12. Carroll SC, Ng SG. Outcomes of orbital blowout fracture surgery in children and adolescents. Br J Ophthalmol 2010;94(6):736–9.

13. Egbert JE, May K, Kersten RC, et al. Pediatric orbital floor fracture : direct extraocular muscle involvement. Ophthalmology 2000;107(10):1875–9.

14. Hatton MP, Watkins LM, Rubin PA. Orbital fractures in children. Ophthalmic Plast Reconstr Surg 2001; 17(3):174–9.

15. Messinger A, Radkowski MA, Greenwald MJ, et al. Orbital roof fractures in the pediatric population. Plast Reconstr Surg 1989;84(2):213–6. discussion 217-8.

16. Moore MH, David DJ, Cooter RD. Oblique craniofacial fractures in children. J Craniofac Surg 1990; 1(1):4–7.

17. Țenț PA, Juncar RI, Moca AE, et al. The Etiology and Epidemiology of Pediatric Facial Fractures in North-Western Romania: A 10-Year Retrospective Study. Children 2022;9(7):932.

18. Zerfowski M, Bremerich A. Facial trauma in children and adolescents. Clin Oral Investig 1998;2(3):120–4.

19. Dufresne C, Manson PN. Pediatric facial injuries. Philadelphia, PA: Saunders Elsevier; 2005. p. 424–34.

20. Rowe NL. Fractures of the facial skeleton in children. J Oral Surg 1968;26(8):505–15.

21. Escaravage GK Jr, Dutton JJ. Age-related changes in the pediatric human orbit on CT. Ophthalmic Plast Reconstr Surg 2013;29(3):150–6.

22. Stricker M, Raphael B, Van der Meulen J, et al. Craniofacial development and growth. Craniofac Malform 1990;61–90.

23. Sperber GH, Sperber SM. Craniofacial development. Beijing: PMPH USA Ltd; 2001.

24. Zimmermann CE, Troulis MJ, Kaban LB. Pediatric facial fractures: recent advances in prevention, diagnosis and management. Int J Oral Maxillofac Surg 2006;35:2–13.

25. Singh DJ, Bartlett SP. Pediatric craniofacial fractures: long-term consequences. Clin Plast Surg 2004;31(3):499–518.

26. Demas PN, Braun TW. Pediatric facial injuries associated with all-terrain vehicles. J Oral Maxillofac Surg 1992;50(12):1280–3.

27. Bartlett SP, DeLozier JB 3rd. Controversies in the management of pediatric facial fractures. Clin Plast Surg 1992;19:245Y258.

28. Martins C, Costa E Silva IE, Campero A, et al. Microsurgical anatomy of the orbit: the rule of seven. Anat Res Int 2011;2011:468727.

29. Fortunato MA, Fielding AF, Guernsey LH. Facial bone fractures in children. Oral Surg Oral Med Oral Pathol 1982;53(3):225–30.

30. Lofgren DH, McGuire D, Gotlib A. Frontal Sinus Fractures. In: StatPearls. Treasure island (FL): StatPearls Publishing; 2022.

31. Sobol DL, Lee A, Susarla SM. Unusual Combined Orbital Roof and Orbital Floor Fractures in A Pediatric Patient. Plast Reconstr Surg Glob Open 2020; 8(12):e3324.

32. Coon D, Yuan N, Jones D, et al. Defining pediatric orbital roof fractures: patterns, sequelae, and indications for operation. Plast Reconstr Surg 2014;134(3): 442e–8e.

33. Kwon JH, Moon JH, Kwon MS, et al. The differences of blowout fracture of the inferior orbital wall between children and adults. Arch Otolaryngol Head Neck Surg 2005;131(8):723–7.

34. De Man K, Wijngaarde R, Hes J, et al. Influence of age on the management of blow-out fractures of the orbital floor. Int J Oral Maxillofac Surg 1991;20: 330Y336.

35. Jordan DR, Allen LH, White J, et al. Intervention within days for some orbital floor fractures: the white-eyed blowout. Ophthalmic Past Reconstr Surg 1998;14(6):379–90.

36. Parbhu KC, Galler KE, Li C, et al. Underestimation of soft tissue entrapment by computed tomography in orbital floor fractures in the pediatric population. Ophthalmology 2008;115:1620–5.

37. Lane K, Penne RB, Bilyk JR. Evaluation and management of pediatric orbital fractures in a primary care setting. Orbit 2007;26(3):183–91.

38. Cohen SM, Garrett CG. Pediatric orbital floor fractures: nausea/vomiting as signs of entrapment. Otolaryngol Head Neck Surg 2003;129:43–7.

39. Sires BS, Stanley RB, Levine LM. Oculocardiac reflex caused by orbital floor trapdoor fracture: an indication for urgent repair. Arch Ophthalmol 1998;116: 955–6.

40. Jank S, Emshoff R, Etzeldorfer M, et al. Ultrasound vs computed tomography in the imaging of orbital floor fractures. J Oral Maxillofac Surg 2004;62: 150–4.

41. Lakits A, Prokesch R, Scholda C, et al. Orbital helical computed tomography in the diagnosis and management of eye trauma. Ophthalmology 1999;106: 2330–5.

42. Kolk A, Stimmer H, Klopfer M, et al. High resolution magnetic resonance imaging with an orbital coil as an alternative to computed tomography scan as the primary imaging modality of pediatric orbital fractures. J Oral Maxillofac Surg 2009;67:348–56.

43. Freund M, Hähnel S, Sartor K. The value of magnetic resonance imaging in the diagnosis of orbital floor fractures. Eur Radiol 2002;12(5):1127–33.

44. Jank S, Deibl M, Strobl H, et al. Interrater reliability of sonographic examinations of orbital fractures. Eur J Radiol 2005;54:344–51.

45. American Academy of Ophthalmology. Basic and clinical science course. Section 7: orbit, eyelids, and lacrimal system. San Fransisco: America Academy of Ophthalmology; 2012. p. 104.

46. Liao JC, Elmalem VI, Wells TS, et al. Surgical timing and postoperative ocular motility in type B orbital blowout fractures. Ophthalmic Plast Reconstr Surg 2015;31(1):29–33.

47. Gerbino G, Roccia F, Bianchi FA, et al. Surgical management of orbital trapdoor fracture in a pediatric population. J Oral Maxillofac Surg 2010;68(6):1310–6.

48. Yamanaka Y, Watanabe A, Sotozono C, et al. Impact of surgical timing of postoperative ocular motility in orbital blowout fractures. Br J Ophthalmol 2018; 102(3):398–403.

49. Wang NC, Ma L, Wu SY, et al. Orbital blow-out fractures in children: characterization and surgical outcome. Chang Gung Med J 2010;33(3):313–20.

50. Smith B, Lisman RD, Simonton J, et al. Volkmann's contracture of the extraocular muscles following blowout fracture. Plast Reconstr Surg 1984;74: 200–16.

51. Coon D, Kosztowski M, Mahoney NR, et al. Principles for Management of Orbital Fractures in the Pediatric Population: A Cohort Study of 150 Patients. Plast Reconstr Surg 2016;137(4):1234–40.

52. Burnstine MA. Clinical recommendations for repair of isolated orbital floor fractures: an evidence-based analysis. Ophthalmology 2002;109(7): 1207–13.

53. Yoon KC, Seo MS, Park YG. Orbital trapdoor fracture in children. J Korean Med Sci 2003;18(6):881–5.

54. Broyles JM, Jones D, Bellamy J, et al. Pediatric orbital floor fractures: outcome analysis of 72 children with orbital floor fractures. Plast Reconstr Surg 2015;136:822–8.

55. Bite U, Jackson IT, Forbes GS, et al. Orbital volume measurements in enophthalmos using three-dimensional CT imaging. Plast Reconstr Surg 1985;75(4):502–8.

56. Parsons GS, Mathog RH. Orbital wall and volume relationships. Arch Otolaryngol Head Neck Surg 1988; 114(7):743–7.

57. Kim SM, Jeong YS, Lee IJ, et al. Prediction of the development of late enophthalmos in pure blowout fractures: delayed orbital tissue atrophy plays a major role. Eur J Ophthalmol 2017;27(1):104–8.

58. Wei LA, Durairaj VD. Pediatric orbital floor fractures. J AAPOS 2011;15(2):173–80.

59. Peng MY, Merbs SL, Grant MP, et al. Orbital fracture repair outcomes with preformed titanium mesh implants and comparison to porous polyethylene coated titanium sheets. J Cranio-Maxillo-Fac Surg 2017;45(2):271–4.

60. Kozakiewicz M, Elgalal M, Loba P, et al. Clinical application of 3D pre-bent titanium implants for orbital floor fractures. J Cranio-Maxillo-Fac Surg 2009;37(4):229–34.

61. Ellis E 3rd, Tan Y. Assessment of internal orbital reconstructions for pure blowout fractures: cranial bone grafts versus titanium mesh. J Oral Maxillofac Surg 2003;61(4):442–53.

62. Abumanhal M, Ben-Cnaan R, Feldman I, et al. Polyester Urethane Implants for Orbital Trapdoor Fracture Repair in Children. J Oral Maxillofac Surg 2019;77(1):126–31.

63. Eppley BL. Use of resorbable plates and screws in pediatric facial fractures. J Oral Maxillofac Surg 2005;63:385–91.

64. Hollier LH, Rogers N, Berzin E, et al. Resorbable mesh in the treatment of orbital floor fractures. J Craniofac Surg 2001;12:242–6.

65. Gerber B, Kiwanuka P, Dhariwal D. Orbital fractures in children: a review of outcomes. Br J Oral Maxillofac Surg 2013;51:789–93.

66. Appling WD, Patrinely JR, Salzer TA. Transconjunctival approach vs subciliary skin-muscle flap approach for orbital fracture repair. Arch Otolaryngol Had Neck Surg 1993;19:1000–7.

67. Patel PC, Sobota BT, Patel NM, et al. Comparison of transconjunctival versus subciliary approaches for orbital fractures: a review of 60 cases. J Craniomaxillofac Trauma 1998;4:17–21.

68. Badakere A, Patil-Chhablani P. Orbital Apex Syndrome: A Review. Eye Intracranial 2019;11:63–72.

69. Stotland MA, Do NK. Pediatric orbital fractures. J Craniofac Surg 2011;22:1230–5.

70. Gagnon MR, Yeatts RP, Williams Z, et al. Delayed enophthalmos following a minimally displaced orbital floor fracture. Ophthalmic Plast Reconstr Surg 2004;20(3):241–3.

71. Lorenz HP, Longaker MT, Kawamoto HK Jr. Primary and secondary orbit surgery: the transconjunctival approach. Plast Reconstr Surg 1999;103(4):1124–8.

72. Rohrich RJ, Janis JE, Adams WP Jr. Subciliary versus subtarsal approaches to orbitozygomatic fractures. Plast Reconstr Surg 2003;111(5):1708–14.

73. Ridgway EB, Chen C, Colakoglu S, et al. The incidence of lower eyelid malposition after facial fracture repair: a retrospective study and meta-analysis comparing subtarsal, subciliary, and transconjunctival incisions. Plast Reconstr Surg 2009; 124(5):1578–86.

74. Wolfe SA, Ghurani R, Podda S, et al. An examination of posttraumatic, postsurgical orbital deformities: conclusions drawn for improvement of primary treatment. Plast Reconstr Surg 2008;122:1870–81.

Pediatric Cranial Vault and Skull Base Fractures

Malia McAvoy, MD, MS[a,b], Richard A. Hopper, MD, MS[a,b], Amy Lee, MD[a,b], Richard G. Ellenbogen, MS, MD[a,b], Srinivas M. Susarla, DMD, MD, MPH[a,b],*

KEYWORDS

- Pediatric skull fracture • Pediatric craniofacial trauma • Pediatric skull base
- Cerebrospinal fluid leakage • Pediatric cranial vault development

KEY POINTS

- Growth and development of the pediatric cranial vault and skull base play a significant role in the patterns of injury seen in pediatric craniofacial trauma.
- The cranial vault grows in a cephalocaudal vector, with 95% of growth completed by age 5.
- Most pediatric vault and skull base fractures can be treated conservatively. Surgical repair may be indicated for fronto-basilar injuries with associated cerebrospinal fluid leak, depressed skull fractures, orbital roof and sphenoid wing fractures, and growing skull fractures.

INTRODUCTION

Head trauma in the pediatric population is extremely common, accounting for 600,000 emergency department visits annually among American children with an incidence of 250 per 100,000 per year.[1] Among all children with head injuries, skull fractures are identified up to 30% of patients. Most pediatric skull fractures can be managed conservatively. Of those requiring surgical intervention, fewer than half of surgeries are performed for skull fracture repair only.[2] Surgical intervention on initial injury is largely performed in cases of skull fracture depression, underlying hemorrhage/mass lesion, frontal or basilar injury with venous sinus involvement or cerebrospinal fluid (CSF) leak. Frontal bone fractures with depression, CSF leak, or cortical injury is the most likely to require repair.[2]

Although the pediatric skull has the advantage over the adult skull of improved capacity to remodel and heal, the developing skull places unique challenges such as growing skull fractures (GSFs) and the essential role of the anterior cranial base in orbital development. This article discusses the normal development of the cranial vault, the role of surgical treatment of pediatric skull fractures and its technical challenges even for experienced multidisciplinary teams.

NORMAL DEVELOPMENT OF THE CRANIAL VAULT

A thorough understanding of normal growth and development of the pediatric skull base and craniofacial structures is important to understand skull fracture patterns. In contrast to the midface (eg, maxilla, zygoma, and nasal complex), and lower face (mandible), cranial vault growth is largely complete by the time children reach mixed dentition.[3]

Craniomaxillofacial growth follows a cephalocaudal vector such that the cranial vault and upper face are relatively prominent in infants and small children (**Fig. 1**A).[3,4] Enlow discusses 2 main morphologic events that direct craniofacial growth including (1) basal cranium growth and (2) development of pharyngeal and facial airway structures.[4] The first phase occurs as a response to rapid growth of the brain and orbit during the first year of life resulting in growth of the cranium, orbit, and upper third of the face.

a Department of Neurosurgery; b Division of Plastic Surgery, Department of Surgery, University of Washington School of Medicine, Craniofacial Center, Seattle Children's Hospital, Seattle, WA, USA
* Corresponding author. Craniofacial Center, Seattle Children's Hospital, 4800 Sand Point Way NE, Seattle, WA 98015.
E-mail address: SRINIVAS.SUSARLA@SEATTLECHILDRENS.ORG

Oral Maxillofacial Surg Clin N Am 35 (2023) 597–606
https://doi.org/10.1016/j.coms.2023.04.008
1042-3699/23/© 2023 Elsevier Inc. All rights reserved.

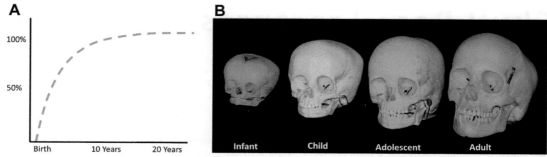

Fig. 1. (*A*) As a result of rapid growth of the cranial vault relative to the midface and mandible, the cranium to facial ratio is approximately 8:1 at birth, 4:1 at age 5 and 2:1 at adolescence. The relative prominence of the upper face relative to the midface and lower face contributes to a greater frequency of cranial vault fractures in infants and small children relative to older children and adults. (*B*) Cranial vault growth velocity over time. The cranial vault grows rapidly in the first few years of life, with 80% to 85% of growth completed by age 2% and 95% of growth completed by age 5.

The cranium is composed of the chondrocranium and the neurocranium. The chondrocranium, or the cranial base, is initially formed as a cartilage model from occipital somites, which eventually becomes bone by endochondral ossification. During the first few months of life, there is progressive ossification of the cribiform plate, roof of the nasal cavities, and crista galli.[5] These ossification centers form the bones of the base of the skull including occipital, sphenoid, temporal, and ethmoid bones. Most growth of the cranial base occurs at articulations called synchondroses. The most significant synchondrosis is called the spheno-occipital synchondrosis, which remains patent until teenage years. Once ossified, the bone can also grow via remodeling, a process called appositional growth. Before the age of 4 years, the anterior skull base is not completely ossified. Normal variant lucencies in the pediatric skull base can be confused for traumatic injuries, so experienced clinical expertise is required in the initial evaluation.

The neurocranium, or cranial vault, is made up of curved, flat bones formed intramembranously from neural crest cells. The growth of these bones occurs at the fibrous articulations, or the sutures. Appositional growth also occurs on the endocortical and ectocortical surfaces. The growth velocity of the cranial vault is rapid in the first few years of life and plateaus between 5 and 7 years of age.[6] Measurement of head circumferences shows that 86% of growth occurs within the first year and 94% of growth within 5 years of age (**Fig. 1**B).

Knowledge of normal paranasal sinus development also guides management of cranial fractures in children.[5] Frontal sinus fracture is not an issue for children who have not yet developed aeration of the frontal air cells. The frontal sinus is the last

of the paranasal sinuses to develop, coming from the anterior ethmoid air cells. Earliest frontal sinus pneumatization occurs at the age of 2. By 4 years of age, the frontal sinus reaches half the height of the orbit, and by 10 years of age, the frontal sinuses extend into the frontal bone.[7]

The development of the orbital wall influences the types of fractures seen in young children. Infants typically have relative frontal bossing, which protects the orbital structures but results in orbital roof fractures being more common than orbital floor fractures in younger aged children.[8] Isolated orbital fractures are relatively rare in children younger than age 5. The frequency of orbital floor fractures does not exceed upper orbit fractures until after age 7.[9]

TYPES OF SKULL FRACTURES

The patterns of skull fractures in older children and adolescents are frequently identical to those found in adults (**Figs. 2–6**). However, the patterns of craniofacial injuries in younger children differ from those in adults, primarily reflecting changes in anatomy and physiology of the developing skull as well as extent of sinus pneumatization.

The location of the fracture on the skull determines treatment strategy. Parietal bone fractures are the most common fracture managed nonoperatively. Frontal bone fractures are more likely to require surgical intervention. These fractures are more likely to involve the frontal sinus, skull base, and orbit as well as have an increased chance of causing a CSF leak, ocular complications, cortical contusion, and cosmetic deformity. Children with aerated frontal sinuses are at higher risk of requiring surgical repair. Other fractures that are more likely to require surgical management

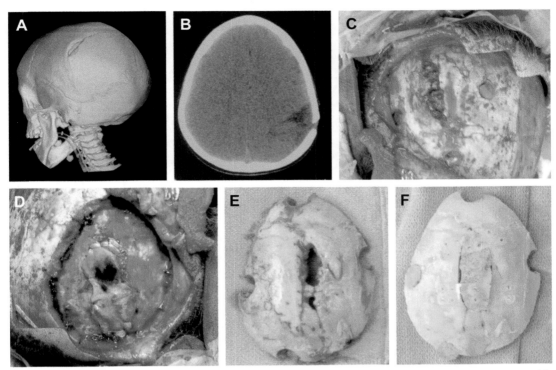

Fig. 2. Growing skull fracture. A growing skull fracture can occur when a dural injury occurs in conjunction with a depressed skull fracture. GSFs represent <1% of skull fractures and are most commonly seen in the first 3 years of life because this is the period of rapid growth of the cranial vault. Clinically, patients will present with a progressively widening soft spot in the site of a prior skull fracture, which may develop within months of the initial injury but not be evident until years later. Imaging will demonstrate a widened bony gap at the site of a prior fracture (*A*), often with evidence of prior brain injury underlying the defect (*B*). Surgical repair involves a craniotomy access the injured dura (*C*), dural repair (*D*), and autologous cranioplasty with split calvarial graft (*E, F*).

include depressed skull fractures (DSFs), orbital fractures, and GSFs.

Growing Skull Fractures

Children aged younger 3 years with skull fractures are at risk of developing diastatic enlargement of the fracture line as brain growth proceeds.[10–12] This phenomenon is called a growing skull fracture (GSF). In a series of 897 pediatric patients with skull fractures, only 1 patient (0.1%) developed a growing fracture requiring a delayed repair.[2] GSF is thought to result from a dural tear through which the leptomeninges and brain parenchyma herniate. This forms a cystic sac, which manifests as a soft, nontender swelling at the site of the fracture.[13,14] Surgery is recommended in almost all cases and involves dural repair with or without cranioplasty.[11,15,16] Early surgical intervention is recommended, regardless of the GSF location, to yield a good cosmetic result and cortical integrity.[11,17] Delay in repair of GSF can result in seizures and focal neurologic deficits.[11,12,15,16]

Skull Base Fractures

Fracture of the skull base may involve several bones such as temporal, occipital, sphenoidal, and spheno-ethmoidal complex as well as orbital portion of the frontal bone. The most common skull base fracture is temporal bone fracture. Skull base fractures may cause associated injuries such as hearing loss, facial nerve injury, and CSF leak.

Dural tears leading to CSF leak are common among skull base fractures due to tight adherence between the skull base and dura, especially in the anterior skull base fractures. The clinical signs of a skull base fracture include retroauricular and/or periorbital bruising, hemotympanum, CSF otorrhea, and rhinorrhea. Dural tears leading to CSF leak are common among skull base fractures due to tight adherence between the skull base and dura, especially in the anterior skull base fractures.[18,19] Most traumatic CSF leaks resolve spontaneously within 1 week. CSF leakage in the setting of a temporal bone fracture ceases more often spontaneously compared with a CSF leak

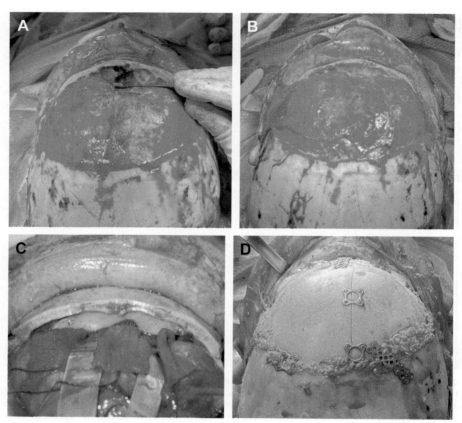

Fig. 3. Anterior cranial base injury with associated CSF leak (*A*). Fronto-basilar fractures in children, in whom the frontal sinus is not developed or incompletely developed, may result in CSF leak. Surgical repair is accomplished via a bifrontal craniotomy, with dural repair. Pedicled pericranial flaps are useful for creating a vascularized barrier between the nasal cavity and subfrontal space (*B*). Small anterior skull base defects may be reconstructed with particulate graft. Larger defects may require cortical grafts, which can be rigidly fixated to the sphenoid wings (*C*). In patients with associated frontal bone injuries, cranioplasty is frequently required (*D*).

associated with the fracture of the anterior cranial fossa.[18]

Surgical repair is required for persistent CSF leaks. Untreated CSF leakage may lead to meningitis, hydrocephalus, subdural fluid collections, and neurocognitive abnormalities. Meningitis develops among 10% to 27.5% of these patients and is associated mortality rate of up to 10%.[18,20] Persistent CSF leak may be managed either by diversion via lumbar drainage or with

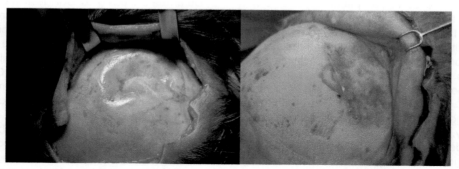

Fig. 4. In infants and young children, the relatively thin bone of the calvarium can result in "ping-pong" type DSFs (left). These are typically treated with craniotomy and autologous cranioplasty (right).

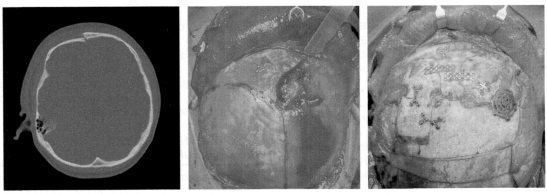

Fig. 5. Depressed skull fracture. As the bone thickens with calvarial development, high-energy injuries can result in DSFs (left, middle), frequently with associated brain injury. Repair frequently requires craniotomy, dural repair, and autologous cranioplasty (right).

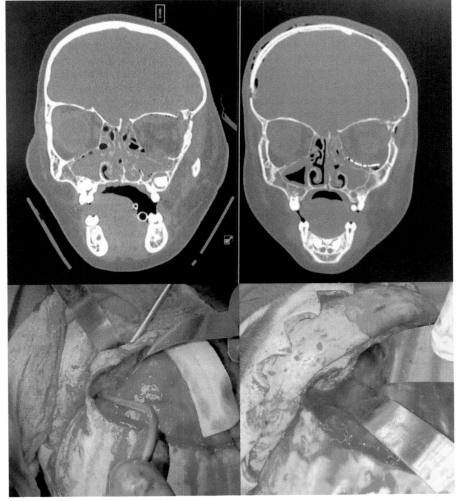

Fig. 6. Orbital roof "blow-in" fractures are frequently seen in small children following trauma to the supraorbital rim, typically resulting in a decrease in orbital volume (top left). Repair is focused on elevating the depressed orbital roof (top right) to restore orbital volume. In older children, the orbital roof may be reliably reduced via a brow or upper eyelid approach. In younger children and those with associated fronto-basilar or intracranial injuries, an intracranial approach may be required (bottom). An uncorrected, displaced orbital roof fracture can result in secondary dystopia, which may require complex orbital movements (eg, box osteotomies) for correction.

extracranial repair.[21] In a series of 63 pediatric patients with skull base fractures, 25% of patients required operative treatment with intracranial, extracranial, or combined approach.[22]

Depressed Skull Fractures

Most isolated nondepressed linear skull fractures can be managed conservatively, and numerous studies have favored discharge rather than observation for these patients.[23–27] Depressed skull fractures (DSFs) DSFs are more likely to be associated with intracranial pathologic condition and morbidity.[2,28] DSFs account for 15% to 25% of children with skull fractures. The term "compound fractures" is used to described contaminated skull fractures where the skin integrity is impaired. In a series of 530 pediatric patients with DSFs, 66% had compound fractures.[29] Compound fractures were more likely to be associated with underlying brain injury than simple fractures alone.

One subtype of DSFs occurring in young children is so called "ping-pong" fractures (see **Fig. 4**).[30] This subtype of DSF occurs when the skull is relatively soft and able to indent without a break in the bone. Ping-pong fractures occur in newborns and young infants and have been reported to spontaneously elevate with growth of the skull, particularly among newborns after birth trauma.[31–33] In general, select DSFs may be managed conservatively except in cases of underlying intracranial hematoma, severe cosmetic defects, compound fractures, and in cases where the bone depression is greater than 1 cm and are associated with cortical deformation (see **Fig. 5**).

Orbital Roof and Sphenoid Fractures

Orbital roof fractures are more common among children than adults. Orbital fractures in children represent a unique subset of fractures with the risk of adjacent intracranial injury. These fractures can also result in entrapment of orbital soft tissues even without significant displacement of the fracture.[5]

There is also the potential for sequelae not seen with fractures elsewhere in the orbit such as pulsatile proptosis and encephaloceles leading to "growing" roof fractures.[34] Similar to GSFs as described previously, the orbitocranial variant of GSF involves herniation of tissue through the fracture line. Due to their proximity to the globe, these injuries can cause proptosis, which may lead to amblyopia in infants.[11,35–37]

Orbitocranial GSFs are associated with specific visual and cosmetic complications as well as the risk of CSF rhinorrhea through communications with the ethmoid sinus.

Fractures of the greater sphenoid wing, including the lateral orbital wall, can result in decreased orbital volume, with associated proptosis and/or vision changes. These fractures frequently require surgical repair to prevent orbital dystopia and, in cases of acute vision compromise, decompression of the globe.

SURGICAL MANAGEMENT
Growing Skull Fracture

The basic surgical principal in the management of GSFs is to repair the defects in both the dura and the cranium (see **Fig. 2**).[11,16,17,34] Liu and colleagues argued that duraplasty alone may suffice in GSF with cranial defects less than 3 cm. Cranioplasty is required for larger defects to prevent recurrence.[16] The procedure involves raising the craniotomy flap around the defect, resecting the herniated dural sac, gently repositioning the herniated cortex in the cranium, followed by watertight dural closure and cranioplasty. Duraplasty may be useful as the dural edges often retract following a tear. Pericranial graft or temporalis fascia may be used for repair.

Skull Base Fracture with Cerebrospinal Fluid Leak

The coronal flap approach provides excellent extracranial exposure for the repair of anterior skull base CSF leaks (see **Fig. 3**). A robust pericranial flap should be harvested at the time of the coronal approach. This flap is utilized to line the skull base and occlude the nasofrontal recess.

Surgical management of frontal sinus fractures involves techniques such as repair (open reduction and internal fixation of the anterior table), obliteration (ablation), and cranialization.[38] A standard coronal incision may be used for all these techniques. The goal of repair of the frontal sinuses is to preserve the sinus anatomy including the nasofrontal duct, sinus mucosa, and anterior and posterior tables. The anterior table is reduced and then stabilized with titanium or resorbable plates and screws. Obliteration involves eliminating the frontal sinus cavity while maintaining the anterior and posterior tables. This technique involves the removal of the anterior table followed by meticulous removal of all mucosa as well as the inner cortex of the sinus wall and the occlusion of the frontonasal duct.

Frontal sinus cranialization is similar to obliteration but the posterior table is removed instead of the anterior table. Often, the frontal sinuses may be cranialized, which means removing the bony wall between the skull's posterior table and opposing dura through an existing frontal bone fracture. However, sometimes this technique

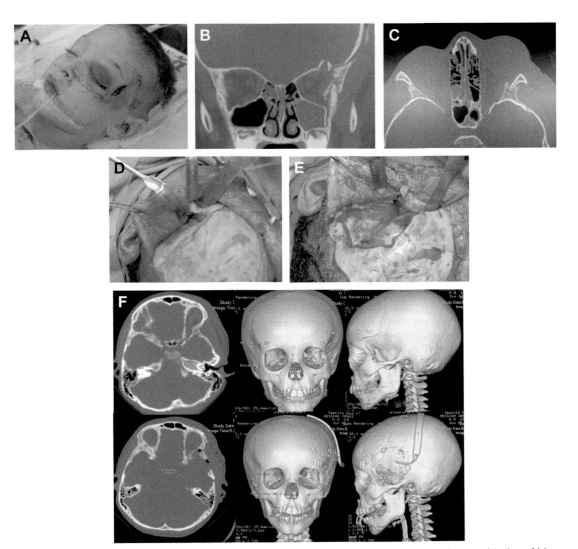

Fig. 7. Spheno-orbital fractures may occur with blows to the lateral orbital wall (*A*). Similar to orbital roof blow-in fractures, these injuries decrease the volume of the orbit, as the lateral orbital wall is pushed inward (*B, C*). Patients may present with proptosis; urgent repair is indicated in patients with vision changes. Repair typically requires a fronto-temporal craniotomy (*D, E*). Successful repair will reconstitute the orbital volume (*F*, top–preoperative; bottom–postoperative).

requires a frontal craniotomy to approach the posterior table. This technique also allows repair of dural lacerations and the ability to attend to any underlying hemorrhage. A pericranial flap is rotated into the defect to isolate the cranium from the frontal sinus. The obstructed duct is sealed with fibrin glue. The anterior table is then reconstructed and stabilized with plates and screws.

Depressed Skull Fracture

Standard surgical management of DSFs involves (1) elevation of the depressed bone fragment, (2) removal of free bone fragments driven into the cerebral cortex, (3) repair of dural defects, (4) evacuation of underlying hematoma, and (4) debridement of wound.[39] Titanium mesh and screws may be used for cranial reconstruction in cases where the bone fragments may be contaminated or if the free fragments are unable to be used.[40] Performing an immediate cranioplasty with titanium mesh instead of leaving the bone defect may improve the child's quality of life with low risk of implant-associated complications. In patients with extensive hemicraniectomy defects, secondary alloplastic reconstruction with customized alloplastic implants may be indicated (see **Fig. 8**).

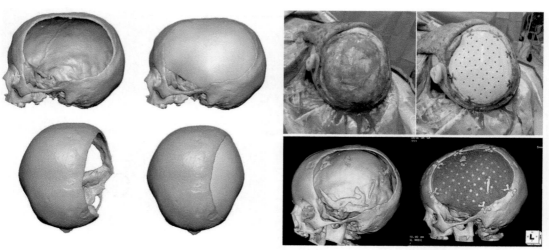

Fig. 8. Children with substantial intracranial injuries requiring decompressive craniectomies will have large hemicraniectomy defects. Although replacement with autologous bone flaps is the standard at most centers, bone flap resorption is not infrequent, due to the magnitude of the associated dural injury and unfavorable environment for graft healing. In situations where bone flap resorption occurs or where the bone flap cannot be utilized due to extensive fracture, alloplastic cranial reconstruction is indicated. Computer-aided design and computer-aided manufacturing processes have dramatically improved the accuracy of reconstructing these complex defects, with an associated decrease in operative time.

Orbital Roof and Sphenoid Fractures

Surgical approaches to orbital roof fractures involve a multidisciplinary team of neurosurgeons, plastic surgeons, and ophthalmologists. Several approaches exist for obtaining access to the anterior skull base for these injuries including a lateral eyebrow incision, upper eyelid incision, and coronal incision. A coronal incision with frontal craniotomy provides wide exposure for dural repair and orbital roof reconstruction (**Figs. 6** and **7**). Reconstruction of the orbit following intracranial exploration and dural closure may be performed using titanium mesh, plates, and screws. Autogenous substances such as calvarium, rib, and ilium can be considered for internal orbital reconstruction but may be difficult to contour to the precise anatomy of the internal orbit and have unpredictable resorption rates.[41]

Secondary Cranial Vault Reconstruction

Cranial reconstruction following a decompressive craniectomy may be achieved by either autologous or synthetic materials. Autologous bone flaps have several advantages over synthetic materials including natural biocompatibility, low risk of rejection, and fit within the original cranial defect without the need for additional contouring.[42–44] Especially in pediatric patients, autologous bone flaps can become reintegrated and grow with the patient.[45,46]

However, the use of autologous bone flaps in the pediatric population has been complicated by high rates of delayed bone resorption (**Fig. 8**).[45] Reintegration of a devascularized bone flap requires a delicate process of revascularization, osteoconduction, osteoinduction, and osteogenesis.[45–47] Any small interferences in this complex process may result in excessive bone resorption. The incidence of cranial bone flap resorption is significantly higher in children ranging between 29.5% and 50%, whereas among adults the incidences range from 3% to 23%.[48–51] Management of bone flap resorption is reconstruction utilizing a synthetic, 3-dimensionally printed implant.

SUMMARY

Although the majority of pediatric skull fractures is nonoperative and may be managed conservatively, the pattern of cranial vault and skull base fractures seen in children varies with their evolving anatomy and requires vigilant management of unique complications, some seen only in the pediatric population. These unique complications are associated with a growing skull and orbital fractures as well as bone flap resorption. The surgical techniques described for the treatment of these fractures are unique and differ compared with the techniques used in adults. Although the surgical repair of skull base fractures may be complex, requiring a multidisciplinary team approach, the spectrum of surgical indications and techniques used are well described in the pediatric and adult literature.

CLINICS CARE POINTS

- Most pediatric vault and skull base fractures can be treated conservatively.

- Surgical repair may be indicated for fronto-basilar injuries with associated CSF leak, DSFs, orbital roof and sphenoid wing fractures, and GSFs.

- In patients with severe brain injuries undergoing decompressive craniectomy autologous cranioplasty is frequently associated with bone resorption. Secondary cranial reconstruction with alloplastic implants is frequently indicated.

REFERENCES

1. Schneier AJ, Shields BJ, Hostetler SG, et al. Incidence of pediatric traumatic brain injury and associated hospital resource utilization in the United States. Pediatrics 2006;118:483–92.
2. Bonfield CM, Naran S, Adetayo OA, et al. Pediatric skull fractures: the need for surgical intervention, characteristics, complications, and outcomes. J Neurosurg Pediatr 2014;14:205–11.
3. Costello BJ, Rivera RD, Shand J, et al. Growth and development considerations for craniomaxillofacial surgery. Oral Maxillofac Surg Clin North Am 2012; 24:377–96.
4. Enlow DH, Kuroda T, Lewis AB. The morphological and morphogenetic basis for craniofacial form and pattern. Angle Orthod 1971;41:161–88.
5. Koch BL. Pediatric considerations in craniofacial trauma. Neuroimaging Clin N Am 2014;24:513–29.
6. Waitzman AA, Posnick JC, Armstrong DC, et al. Craniofacial skeletal measurements based on computed tomography: Part I. Accuracy and reproducibility. Cleft Palate Craniofac J 1992;29:112–7.
7. Scuderi AJ, Harnsberger HR, Boyer RS. Pneumatization of the paranasal sinuses: normal features of importance to the accurate interpretation of CT scans and MR images. AJR Am J Roentgenol 1993;160:1101–4.
8. Cobb AR, Jeelani NO, Ayliffe PR. Orbital fractures in children. Br J Oral Maxillofac Surg 2013;51:41–6.
9. Koltai PJ, Amjad I, Meyer D, et al. Orbital fractures in children. Arch Otolaryngol Head Neck Surg 1995; 121:1375–9.
10. Lende RA, Erickson TC. Growing skull fractures of childhood. J Neurosurg 1961;18:479–89.
11. Prasad GL, Gupta DK, Mahapatra AK, et al. Surgical results of growing skull fractures in children: a single centre study of 43 cases. Childs Nerv Syst 2015;31: 269–77.
12. Tandon PN, Banerji AK, Bhatia R, et al. Cranio-cerebral erosion (growing fracture of the skull in children). Part II. Clinical and radiological observations. Acta Neurochir 1987;88:1–9.
13. Goldstein FP, Rosenthal SA, Garancis JC, et al. Varieties of growing skull fractures in childhood. J Neurosurg 1970;33:25–8.
14. Taveras JM, Ransohoff J. Leptomeningeal cysts of the brain following trauma with erosion of the skull; a study of seven cases treated by surgery. J Neurosurg 1953;10:233–41.
15. Gupta SK, Reddy NM, Khosla VK, et al. Growing skull fractures: a clinical study of 41 patients. Acta Neurochir 1997;139:928–32.
16. Liu XS, You C, Lu M, et al. Growing skull fracture stages and treatment strategy. J Neurosurg Pediatr 2012;9:670–5.
17. Wang X, Li G, Li Q, et al. Early diagnosis and treatment of growing skull fracture. Neurol India 2013;61: 497–500.
18. Friedman JA, Ebersold MJ, Quast LM. Post-traumatic cerebrospinal fluid leakage. World J Surg 2001;25:1062–6.
19. Mendizabal GR, Moreno BC, Flores CC. Cerebrospinal fluid fistula: frequency in head injuries. Rev Laryngol Otol Rhinol 1992;113:423–5.
20. Marentette LJ, Valentino J. Traumatic anterior fossa cerebrospinal fluid fistulae and craniofacial considerations. Otolaryngol Clin North Am 1991;24: 151–63.
21. Bell RB, Dierks EJ, Homer L, et al. Management of cerebrospinal fluid leak associated with craniomaxillofacial trauma. J Oral Maxillofac Surg 2004;62: 676–84.
22. Perheentupa U, Kinnunen I, Grenman R, et al. Management and outcome of pediatric skull base fractures. Int J Pediatr Otorhinolaryngol 2010;74: 1245–50.
23. Arneitz C, Sinzig M, Fasching G. Diagnostic and clinical management of skull fractures in children. J Clin Imaging Sci 2016;6:47.
24. Arrey EN, Kerr ML, Fletcher S, et al. Linear nondisplaced skull fractures in children: who should be observed or admitted? J Neurosurg Pediatr 2015; 16:703–8.
25. Blackwood BP, Bean JF, Sadecki-Lund C, et al. Observation for isolated traumatic skull fractures in the pediatric population: unnecessary and costly. J Pediatr Surg 2016;51:654–8.
26. Bressan S, Marchetto L, Lyons TW, et al. A systematic review and meta-analysis of the management and

outcomes of isolated skull fractures in children. Ann Emerg Med 2018;71:714–724 e712.

27. Donaldson K, Li X, Sartorelli KH, et al. Management of isolated skull fractures in pediatric patients: a systematic review. Pediatr Emerg Care 2019;35:301–8.

28. Adepoju A, Adamo MA. Posttraumatic complications in pediatric skull fracture: dural sinus thrombosis, arterial dissection, and cerebrospinal fluid leakage. J Neurosurg Pediatr 2017;20:598–603.

29. Ersahin Y, Mutluer S, Mirzai H, et al. Pediatric depressed skull fractures: analysis of 530 cases. Childs Nerv Syst 1996;12:323–31.

30. Zia Z, Morris AM, Paw R. Ping-pong fracture. BMJ Case Rep 2009;2009. bcr2006043570.

31. Loeser JD, Kilburn HL, Jolley T. Management of depressed skull fracture in the newborn. J Neurosurg 1976;44:62–4.

32. Ross G. Spontaneous elevation of a depressed skull fracture in an infant. case report. J Neurosurg 1975; 42:726–7.

33. Sorar M, Fesli R, Gurer B, et al. Spontaneous elevation of a ping-pong fracture: case report and review of the literature. Pediatr Neurosurg 2012;48:324–6.

34. Singh V, Sasidharan GM, Bhat DI, et al. Growing skull fracture and the orbitocranial variant: nuances of surgical management. Pediatr Neurosurg 2017; 52:161–7.

35. Caffo M, Germano A, Caruso G, et al. Growing skull fracture of the posterior cranial fossa and of the orbital roof. Acta Neurochir 2003;145:201–8 [discussion: 208].

36. Jamjoom ZA. Growing fracture of the orbital roof. Surg Neurol 1997;48:184–8.

37. Meier JD, Dublin AB, Strong EB. Leptomeningeal cyst of the orbital roof in an adult: case report and literature review. Skull Base 2009;19:231–5.

38. Bell RB. Management of frontal sinus fractures. Oral Maxillofac Surg Clin North Am 2009;21:227–42.

39. Satardey RS, Balasubramaniam S, Pandya JS, et al. Analysis of factors influencing outcome of depressed fracture of skull. Asian J Neurosurg 2018;13:341–7.

40. Hitoshi Y, Yamashiro S, Yoshida A, et al. Cranial reconstruction with titanium mesh for open depressed skull fracture in children: reports of two cases with long-term observation. Kurume Med J 2020;66:77–80.

41. Kim JW, Bae TH, Kim WS, et al. Early reconstruction of orbital roof fractures: clinical features and treatment outcomes. Arch Plast Surg 2012;39:31–5.

42. Fu KJ, Barr RM, Kerr ML, et al. An outcomes comparison between autologous and alloplastic cranioplasty in the pediatric population. J Craniofac Surg 2016;27:593–7.

43. Klieverik VM, Miller KJ, Singhal A, et al. Cranioplasty after craniectomy in pediatric patients-a systematic review. Childs Nerv Syst 2019;35:1481–90.

44. Rocque BG, Amancherla K, Lew SM, et al. Outcomes of cranioplasty following decompressive craniectomy in the pediatric population. J Neurosurg Pediatr 2013;12:120–5.

45. Grant GA, Jolley M, Ellenbogen RG, et al. Failure of autologous bone-assisted cranioplasty following decompressive craniectomy in children and adolescents. J Neurosurg 2004;100:163–8.

46. Lam S, Kuether J, Fong A, et al. Cranioplasty for large-sized calvarial defects in the pediatric population: a review. Craniomaxillofac Trauma Reconstr 2015;8:159–70.

47. Hersh DS, Anderson HJ, Woodworth GF, et al. Bone flap resorption in pediatric patients following autologous cranioplasty. Oper Neurosurg (Hagerstown) 2021;20:436–43.

48. Iwama T, Yamada J, Imai S, et al. The use of frozen autogenous bone flaps in delayed cranioplasty revisited. Neurosurgery 2003;52:591–6 [discussion: 595-596].

49. Malcolm JG, Mahmooth Z, Rindler RS, et al. Autologous cranioplasty is associated with increased reoperation rate: a systematic review and meta-analysis. World Neurosurg 2018;116:60–8.

50. Piedra MP, Thompson EM, Selden NR, et al. Optimal timing of autologous cranioplasty after decompressive craniectomy in children. J Neurosurg Pediatr 2012;10:268–72.

51. Schuss P, Vatter H, Oszvald A, et al. Bone flap resorption: risk factors for the development of a long-term complication following cranioplasty after decompressive craniectomy. J Neurotrauma 2013; 30:91–5.

Pediatric Panfacial Fractures

Sameer Shakir, MD[a],*, Russell E. Ettinger, MD[b,c], Srinivas M. Susarla, DMD, MD, MPH[b,c], Craig B. Birgfeld, MD[b,c]

KEYWORDS

- Panfacial trauma • Pediatric facial fracture • Craniofacial growth

KEY POINTS

- Pediatric craniomaxillofacial trauma differs from that of adults in terms of management, epidemiology, injury pattern, and long-term growth.
- Although pediatric panfacial fractures are rare, they are associated with polytrauma that risks severe morbidity and mortality and requires high-acuity multidisciplinary care.
- The surgical management of pediatric panfacial fractures is generally more conservative not only due to inherently augmented healing and remodeling capacity but also due to concern over future growth impairment.
- Undertreatment of displaced fractures in the pediatric population, however, may lead to deformities in adulthood that are exceedingly challenging to treat secondarily.

INTRODUCTION

Although rare, pediatric panfacial injuries pose significant bony and soft tissue reconstructive challenges owing to anatomic differences and the potential for future growth and development. Manson and colleagues defined panfacial fractures as those involving the upper (frontal bone), middle (midface), and lower (occlusal unit) facial thirds (**Fig. 1**A).[1] Contemporaneous definitions have broadened to include fractures of the midface and mandible because reconstruction follows the same principles as those for a true panfacial fracture (see **Fig. 3**A).[2–4] In pediatric patients, facial trauma often involves the soft tissue or dentoalveolar structures.[5] The presence of multilevel injury is frequently indicative of a high-energy trauma with potential life-threatening consequences that must be appropriately prioritized according to Advanced Trauma Life Support (ATLS) protocols.

Management of pediatric facial fractures is more conservative than that of adults to minimize deleterious effects on future growth and development. In the largest reported series of pediatric panfacial injuries, Dalena and colleagues reported an operative rate of 46% with most patients managed nonoperatively to preserve osteogenic and growth potential.[4] Nevertheless, surgical indications for fracture fixation relate to the presence of displaced fractures. Undertreatment of displaced pediatric fractures often results in exceedingly challenging end-stage deformities encountered at skeletal maturity. Limited soft tissue dissection, autogenous bone grafting, and fixation using titanium or resorbable devices are used to minimize the appearance of premature aging while yielding appropriate anatomical reduction and stable fixation.

Unlike the adult population, operative sequencing of pediatric panfacial fractures may favor a top–down rather than bottom–up approach due to routine conservative management of critical growth centers including the mandibular condyle.[4,6,7] Similar to the adult population, dissection and fixation should extend from stable to unstable regions to appropriately reestablish facial width, height, and projection.

a Division of Plastic Surgery, Children's Wisconsin, Milwaukee, WI, USA; b Department of Surgery, Division of Plastic Surgery, University of Washington, 4800 Sand Point Way NE, M/S OB.9.520, Seattle, WA 98150, USA; c Craniofacial Center, Seattle Children's Hospital, 4800 Sand Point Way NE, M/S OB.9.520, Seattle, WA 98150, USA
* Corresponding author. Plastic Surgery, 9000 West Wisconsin Avenue, Suite 340, Milwaukee, WI 53202.
E-mail address: sashakir@mcw.edu

Oral Maxillofacial Surg Clin N Am 35 (2023) 607–617
https://doi.org/10.1016/j.coms.2023.04.006
1042-3699/23/© 2023 Elsevier Inc. All rights reserved.

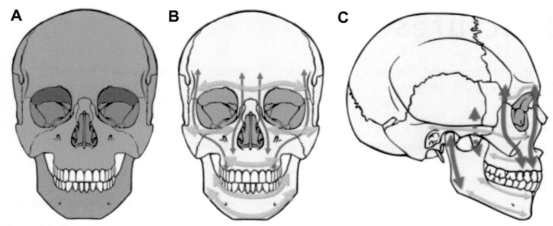

Fig. 1. (*A*) Three bony subunits of the face. Frontal bone and cranium (*blue*), midface (*green*), and mandible (*pink*). The midface consists of the maxilla, zygoma, nasal, lacrimal, ethmoid, and palatine bones. (*B*) Horizontal buttresses (*gold*). Supraorbital bar, infraorbital rims and zygomatic arch, lower maxillary and palate, upper mandibular, and lower mandibular buttresses. (*C*) Vertical buttresses (*purple*). Posterior vertical mandibular, pterygomaxillary, maxillary-zygomatic-frontal, and the medial maxillary naso-frontal buttresses. (*From* Massenburg BB, Lang MS. Management of Panfacial Trauma: Sequencing and Pitfalls. Semin Plast Surg. 2021;35(4):292-298. Published 2021 Sep 23.)

Pediatric Facial Anatomy and Fracture Patterns

The various regions of the craniofacial skeleton achieve skeletal maturity at different times, which correlates with the variable patterns of facial fractures seen in growing children. Upper, middle, and lower facial growth occurs in a cranial to caudal direction from infancy to adolescence. The cranial-to-facial ratio begins at 8:1 at birth with prominent frontal projection and decreases to 2:1 at maturity, which accounts for the comparatively increased incidence of cranial vault fractures and severe head injury observed in the pediatric population.[8] By 2 years of age, the neurocranium has achieved 75% of its growth. By 10 years of age, the neurocranium has achieved 95% of its growth potential, although facial growth lags behind at 65%.[9] Unlike cranial growth, which demonstrates continuous development, facial growth demonstrates discontinuous growth until adolescence.[9] Specifically, facial growth at 3 months approximates 40% of its adult growth potential, 70% at 2 years, and 80% at 5 years. The completion of facial growth subsequently occurs during the pubertal growth spurt.[9] Consequently, facial fractures occurring during the periods of mixed dentition and the pubertal growth spurt may lead to facial asymmetry, particularly if displaced and untreated.

Craniofacial growth centers include cartilage/synchondroses and sutures/periosteum.[10–12] With sinus aeration beginning around 4 to 5 years (as early as 2 years), maturation of the frontal sinus occurs throughout puberty. Underlying brain and ocular signaling determines maturation of the upper face and orbits, with orbital growth typically complete by 6 to 8 years. Maxillary sinus pneumatization correlates with dental development, as the sinus reaches the nasal floor around 12 years when most of the permanent dentition has erupted. The septal midface drives nasomaxillary growth while the condylar growth center dictates posterior height. Alveolar development during eruption of the permanent dentition drives vertical maxillary growth.[5] The mandibular symphysis fused around 2 years, which coincides with the eruption of the primary dentition. Muscle activation signals vertical mandibular growth at the condyles, with bony surface remodeling continuing into puberty.[13] Enlow's theory of apposition and resorption (ie, bony deposition on one side followed by resorption on the other) helps to explain maxillary and mandibular growth.[14] Furthermore, Moss's "functional matrix" theory highlights the importance of the periosteum as a major contributor to bone formation.[10] Applying this conceptual framework to management, subperiosteal exposure of fractures in pediatric patients should be limited only to the extent required to visualize the fracture and apply fixation.

With increasing age, pediatric facial fracture patterns shift in frequency from a cranial to caudal direction. Anatomic factors associated with this change include further development of the midface and mandible and increased bone mineralization, which decreases bony elasticity after age 2 to 3 years.[9] The lack of well-developed facial buttresses results from unerupted dentition, decreased paranasal sinus pneumatization, and increased cancellous bone.[9] Unlike the characteristic LeFort fracture patterns observed in adults, pediatric facial fractures typically present in oblique orientations due to these distinct anatomic differences.[15,16] These obliquely oriented fractures extend across the prominent frontal bone, radiate into the anterior cranial base, and extend across the orbit into the maxilla while typically sparing the mandible.[9,15]

Epidemiology of Pediatric Facial Fractures

Although a detailed epidemiologic overview will be discussed in another article, a brief review is critical to understand the complexities posed by multilevel pediatric facial trauma. In a review of the National Trauma Database, Imahara and colleagues identified 277,008 pediatric trauma patients with 4.6% sustaining facial fractures.[8] The proportion of patients with facial fractures increased with increasing age, suffered from unrestrained blunt trauma (eg, motor vehicle collision [MVC]), and was more likely to be men and Caucasian.[8] Nasal and maxillary fractures were most common in infants, whereas mandible fractures were most common among teenagers. A quarter of patients underwent operative fracture fixation during their initial hospitalization, with increasing age predicting operative management—unsurprisingly, only 11% of toddlers aged 2 to 4 years underwent operative management.[8]

As described above, key anatomical differences help to explain the overall decreased incidence of pediatric facial fractures when compared with adults. Craniofacial disproportion, underdevelopment of the paranasal sinuses, added bimaxillary strength from unerupted dentition, relative micrognathia, well-developed fat pads, compliant sutures, and a viscoelastic skeleton are protective mechanisms unique to the pediatric population.[8,9,17–22] The finding of displaced facial fractures in the pediatric patient consequently suggests a high-energy mechanism and the possibility of severe concomitant injuries outside of the craniofacial skeleton. Based on the Abbreviated Injury Scale, patients with facial fractures demonstrated a 2-fold increase in their Injury Severity Scores, when compared with patients without facial fractures.[8] The prevalence of brain injury, skull base fracture, cervical spine fracture, and blunt cerebrovascular injury were considerably higher among patients found to have facial fractures.[8] Moreover, the facial fracture cohort had a

3-fold increase in intensive care length of stay, 2-fold increase in total length of stay, increased ventilator requirement, and higher mortality rate (4.0 vs 2.5%).[8]

CLINICAL EVALUATION

The increased incidence of severe concomitant injuries to the head and chest that typically accompany pediatric bony trauma necessitates age-appropriate ATLS protocols that prioritize the primary survey and resuscitation while deferring management of potentially "distracting" craniofacial injuries to the secondary survey.[5,23] As head and neck trauma accounts for more than 66% of child abuse, nonaccidental trauma should be suspected if there are inconsistences in the history, prolonged duration between injury and presentation, noncompliance, and/or multiple presentations.[24,25]

Airway management may be challenging in the context of inherently flaccid pharyngeal and anterior laryngeal structures that may be concomitantly injured leading to hypoxia.[5] Associated comminuted mandible fractures may lead to tongue base collapse owing to decreased support of the genioglossus and geniohyoid muscles anteriorly.[3,26] Established mechanisms for airway control including oral intubation, nasal intubation, submental intubation, and tracheostomy.[27] Oral intubation may affect appropriate reduction and fixation of the occlusal unit unless there is the absence of occlusion or absent teeth to allow for posterior placement. Nasal intubation limits comprehensive management of nasal and naso-orbito-ethmoid (NOE) fractures and may be contraindicated in the setting of skull base injury. Submental intubation, which is less morbid than a tracheostomy, allows for the management of complex midface fractures and restoration of the occlusal unit but may be contraindicated in comminuted mandible fractures that require a transcervical approach.[28] Tracheostomy may ultimately be indicated to secure a stable airway away from extensive craniomaxillofacial injury, however, carries its own complication profile.[27]

Arterial bleeding may be present from wounds involving the scalp, tongue, and/or nose. Large scalp wounds may be temporarily controlled with staples or tacking sutures while the nasal passages may be packed with intranasal gauze or Foley catheters to tamponade anterior nasal bleeding. Posterior midface bleeding may require prompt interventional embolotherapy.[29] Hypotension and hypothermia are inherent risks for the pediatric polytrauma patient in the setting of increased cardiopulmonary compensation despite significant blood loss and increased body surface

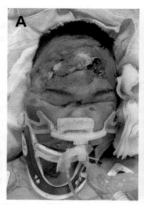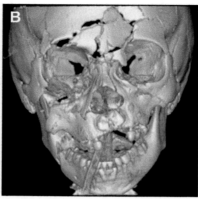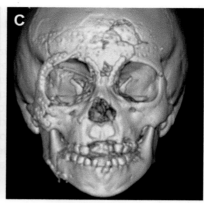

Fig. 2. (*A*) Traditional panfacial presentation. A 5-year-old boy involved in an all terrain vehicle (ATV) rollover presenting with panfacial fractures. Secondary survey is notable for a large transverse full-thickness forehead laceration with open, comminuted fractures of the frontal bone. (*B*) Preoperative CT imaging. Underlying fractures include comminuted, displaced frontal bone fractures, severely displaced right LeFort 1/2/3 fractures, mild-to-moderately displaced left LeFort 2 fracture, and severely displaced right mandibular body fracture with malocclusion. (*C*) Immediate postoperative fracture fixation. Through a top–down, outside–in approach, he underwent ORIF of his bifrontal bone fractures using a resorbable plating system followed by titanium fixation of the right zygoma and the bilateral NOE segments. Following established of midface width and projection, he underwent upper titanium fixation of his right maxilla along the zygomaticomaxillary "buttress" to restore midfacial height through an upper sulcus intraoral approach. Finally, he underwent titanium fixation of the right mandibular body using monocortical fixation along the inferior border through an extraoral approach to control for lingual splay. The remaining nondisplaced and mildly displaced fractures were allowed to heal and remodel.

area:volume ratio.[5] As previously discussed, the increased risk for intracranial, ocular, and cervical spine injuries highlights the importance of prompt neurosurgical and ophthalmologic evaluation to preserve brain, vision, and hearing function. In infants and toddlers, the cervical spine should be carefully supported despite radiographic clearance given their increased cranial-to-facial ratios and increased cartilaginous component of the vertebral column.[24] Periorbital fractures and injuries with concern for visual loss should be promptly evaluated by ophthalmology.

Physical examination should include assessment of characteristic signs and patterns suggestive of underlying fractures such as hypertelorism, Battle sign, malocclusion, trismus, entrapment, periorbital ecchymoses, paresthesia, otorrhea, and rhinorrhea (**Fig. 2**A).[24] Computed tomography (CT) imaging serves as a critical diagnostic and surgical planning tool especially for maxillofacial fractures that may be greensticked or nondisplaced (**Fig. 2**B). High-dose CT imaging risks the development of cataracts, whereas low-dose CT imaging compromises visualization of the overlying soft tissues and intracranial structures.[5] Plain film radiography may be of limited value in fracture detection due to distinct pediatric anatomy including developing tooth buds and nonpneumatized sinuses, for example.[30–32] In panfacial trauma, a systemic review of imaging in a top–

down approach, for example, helps to ensure identification the full catalog of facial injuries.

Sequencing

Unlike the adult population where fracture fixation may be delayed within 7 to 14 days of injury in the setting of prohibitive localized edema, malunion may develop within 3 to 4 days of injury given the enhanced healing potential of pediatric patients.[24] In the setting of panfacial injuries, reconstructive principles include (1) preservation of brain, vision, and hearing function; (2) stabilization of open mandible fractures; (3) provisional skeletal support until definitive reconstruction; (4) preservation of the soft tissues including neurovascular and ductal elements, cranial nerves, and lacrimal system; (5) systematic fracture fixation planning; (6) limited bone grafting in the setting of precise sequential fracture reduction; and (7) soft tissue reconstruction.[29] In general, panfacial injuries compromise the relationship between the occlusal unit and skull base with a loss of customary structures needed for anatomic alignment (**Fig. 1**B, C).[2] Gruss and colleagues popularized the top–down/outside–in approach, which begins with establishing facial width along the frontal bar and cranial base articulation (**Fig. 2**A–C).[33] This approach serves as the historical preference for plastic surgeons owing to their comparative comfort with establishing facial width and projection.[34] Markowitz and Manson popularized the bottom–up/inside–out approach, which focuses first on the occlusal unit and has been championed by oral and maxillofacial surgeons.[29,35–37] Often, patient presentation will dictate one approach over the other in the setting of significant comminution of the occlusal unit or cranial bone, for example.

Operative considerations include working from stable bone to unstable bone, adequate sequential bony reduction of displaced fractures, avoiding unnecessary grafting of malreduced segments, and careful autologous bone grafting of severely comminuted or missing bone.[3] Autologous bone grafting may be obtained from the iliac crest, rib, or cranium.[38] Incision patterns follow standard approaches utilized in the adult population in addition to utilization or extension of preexisting lacerations. Additional pediatric considerations include conservative treatment of greenstick-type fractures owing to a comparatively increased periosteum-to-bone ratio, iatrogenic injury to growth centers from extensive periosteal stripping, growth suture restriction from rigid fixation, and evolving scar formation.[5,39]

Top–down/outside–in approach

Cranium and orbital roof Existing scalp lacerations or a formal coronal incision may be used to access the fronto-orbital region. Goals of frontal bone management include correcting the cranial contour especially along the supraorbital ridge, adequate fracture reduction with relation to other cranial bones, and management of cerebrospinal fluid (CSF) leak. The pediatric cranium, which is more elastic than the mature bicortical skull, can develop "ping pong" or nondisplaced linear fractures that are challenging to identify and treat.[5] These fracture types, as well as growing skull fractures, are covered elsewhere in this volume.

Interestingly, children who sustain significant trauma to the frontal/glabellar region may develop hypoplasia of the frontal sinus—as seen in patients who undergo fronto-orbital reconstruction for craniosynostosis in infancy.[39,40] Although nondisplaced fractures do not require operative fixation, displaced fractures or underlying injuries to the nasofrontal ducts require reduction and fixation. After the frontal sinus has pneumatized, operative management mirrors the algorithmic approach utilized in the adult population.[41] Before frontal sinus aeration, direct cranial trauma may propagate along the orbital roof toward the orbital apex, resulting in injury to the optic nerve, dura mater, and brain with associated hypoglobus, proptosis, gaze restriction, and pulsatile exophthalmos.[5,42] Associated intracranial injury, bony fragment impingement, and ocular findings (eg, exophthalmos, mechanical gaze restriction, lid ptosis, ophthalmoplegia, and vision loss) warrant surgical repair in the form of open reduction and fixation or removal and replacement with autologous bone via a coronal approach and bifrontal craniotomy.[5,43] An anteriorly based pericranial flap may be utilized to reinforce an underlying dural repair if there is any concern for CSF leak.

Zygoma and Orbit

Once the fronto-orbital frame has been reestablished, the zygomatic body and arches are reduced to narrow the facial width, correct orbital dystopia, and restore appropriate malar projection. Displaced zygoma fractures may be managed similarly to the adult population with the caveat of avoiding fixation-related damage to unerupted maxillary dentition. Consequently, fixation can be limited to the superior portions of the zygomaticomaxillary complex in the setting of increased capacity for pediatric bony remodeling (see **Fig. 2**C).[5] Inadequate reduction of the facial width results in a commonly observed broad, flat facial appearance in panfacial injuries.

Orbital floor fractures in children occur following pneumatization of the maxillary sinuses.[39] Fractures with true extraocular muscle entrapment warrant urgent treatment within 8 hours to prevent critical muscle ischemia, Volkmann's type contracture, and subsequent motility issues, which can portend a need for strabismus surgery.[44,45] Unlike the adult population, entrapment of the periorbita results from increased elasticity and greenstick-type fractures observed in pediatric patients. The mechanism involves blunt ocular trauma that transiently increases intraocular pressure and temporarily displaces the orbital floor into the maxillary sinus. The inferior periorbital tissues subsequently herniate into the maxillary sinus. Once the intraocular pressure normalizes, the displaced orbital floor returns to its anatomic alignment, leaving the periorbita/inferior rectus muscle trapped within the sinus.[5,39] Orbital entrapment remains a clinical diagnosis with examination findings including extraocular movement restriction, diplopia, increased scleral show of the contralateral eye during upward gaze (ie, "white eye fracture"), and oculocardiac reflex with vagally mediated symptoms including nausea, vomiting, bradycardia, and hypotension.[5] Reconstruction can be performed through a transconjunctival or transcutaneous incision as part of panfacial fracture exposure. Following reduction of the periorbital contents, autologous bone graft from the iliac crest, rib, or cranium (eg, split cranial bone graft or pericranial shave graft) may be used for orbital floor reconstruction.[5,45] Recently, resorbable alloplastic materials have demonstrated equal efficacy when compared with autologous grafts.[46]

Naso-Orbito-Ethmoid and Nasoseptum

Once the upper, outer bony support (ie, frontozygomatic) has been established, the medial vertical buttress can be restored. NOE fractures account for less than 1% of pediatric facial fractures but present significant reconstructive challenges as a significant portion of patients ultimately require revision to restore appropriate projection of the nasal dorsum and correct secondary telecanthus.[9] Similar to the adult population, NOE fractures are classified and treated according to the same Markowitz system.[5,8,47] Lopez and colleagues proposed nonoperative management of Type I fractures, case-by-case operative management of Type II fractures depending on the presence of permanent dentition, degree of displacement, and presence of open fracture, and consistent operative management of Type III fractures with transnasal wiring, canthal barb resuspension, or suture canthopexy.[5,48]

The increased cartilaginous composition, bony elasticity, and decreased dorsal projection of the pediatric nose results in relative protection of the nasoseptal unit when compared with the adult population.[5] However, this increased deforming capacity results in increased septal distortion and increased risk of hematoma, which must be promptly drained to prevent abscess and saddle-nose deformity. When possible, nonoperative or closed reduction of nasoseptal fractures should be performed due to the septum's role as a critical growth center. Nevertheless, severe injuries of the central midface result in the loss of nasoglabellar support that benefit from open reduction and/or reconstruction in the form of dorsal nasal cantilever bone grafting to restore adequate projection.[3,49]

Occlusal Unit

Following central midface reconstruction, the remaining panfacial injuries relate to the occlusal unit (**Fig. 3**B, C). Unerupted maxillary dentition and the lack of maxillary sinus pneumatization in patients aged younger than 5 years provide relative protection against maxillary fractures. Similar to adult reconstructive principles, the medial and lateral maxillary buttresses should be restored through reduction and/or judicious autologous bone grafting if needed. Iatrogenic growth disturbances can be avoided by limiting subperiosteal

dissection and appreciating future dental compensation in patients presenting with injuries during the period of mixed dentition.[5] In severely displaced fractures requiring open reduction and internal fixation, patients should be counseled on future growth impairment in the form of nasomaxillary hypoplasia telecanthus, and/or vertical growth deficiency.[50]

Once the maxillary width is restored, a palatal split may be fixated using hardware or a prefabricated splint based on the preinjury arch width. Interdental fixation remains a challenge in the pediatric population and securing wires may need to pass around the zygomatic arch or piriform through the palate using a passing trocar to avoid injury to primary or developing dentition.[5] If there is significant maxillary comminution or easier access to the mandible, maxillary reconstruction can be deferred until after mandible fixation. Alternatively, lower midface fractures may be allowed to heal with an understanding that expectant malocclusion, tooth loss, and/or contour irregularities will require subsequent orthognathic surgery, osteointegrated implants, and onlay grafting/alloplastic reconstruction.[39] Proponents of this approach cite the cleft literature, which documents undergrowth of the maxilla in the setting of periosteal elevation of the hard palate.[51]

Assuming prior fixation of the midface with restoration of the maxillary width, the mandible can then be placed into alignment. The presence of developing tooth buds and increased bony elasticity results in pediatric mandible fractures that are typically nondisplaced or mildly displaced. Growth centers located along the condyles, posterior border of the ramus, and dentoalveolus favor conservative management of pediatric mandible fractures, given their remarkable remodeling capacity (**Fig. 3**D, E). Mild malocclusion may resolve spontaneously with eruption of the permanent dentition and subsequent remodeling with growth. Consequently, minimally-to-mildly displaced pediatric mandible fractures may be reasonably managed with observation and a soft, nonchew diet.[5] With the top–down/outside–in approach, open fixation of a mandibular condylar fracture can be avoided, which is especially important in the growing mandible. Injury to the condyle, whether posttraumatic or iatrogenic, can lead to growth arrest and temporomandibular joint bony ankylosis, resulting in retrognathia, facial asymmetry, malocclusion, and limited mouth opening.[39] Several studies have demonstrated reasonable results concerning subsequent growth following conservative treatment.[52,53] Stratifying by dentition, Lopez and colleagues suggested nonoperative management of condylar fractures in the

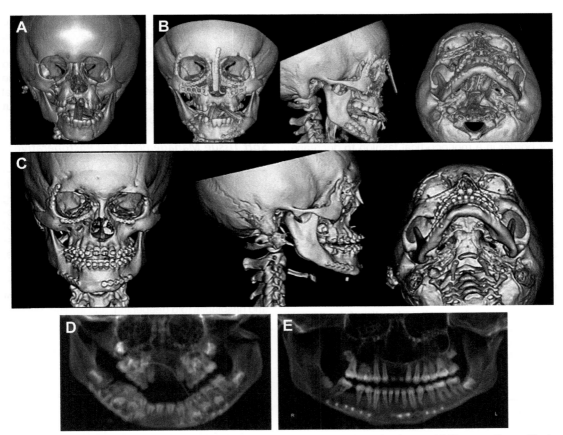

Fig. 3. (*A*) Contemporaneous panfacial presentation. A 6-year-old girl involved in an MVC presenting with significant injuries to the occlusal unit while sparing the frontobasilar region. Preoperative CT imaging is notable for displaced bilateral LeFort 1/2/3 fractures and 4-piece mandible with severely displaced right body, minimally displaced left parasymphysis, and displaced left subcondylar fractures. (*B*) Immediate postoperative fracture fixation. Through a top–down, outside–in approach, she underwent open reduction and internal fixation (ORIF) of bilateral zygoma fractures from to restore facial width followed by bilateral orbital floor reconstruction using titanium mesh implants to correct orbital dystopia and ORIF of bilateral NOE fractures with cantilever reconstruction of the nasal dorsum using split cranial bone graft to restore central midfacial projection. Next, she underwent spanning ladder plate reconstruction of the maxilla from the zygomatic body to the nasomaxillary buttresses to restore midfacial weight and set the midfacial height. Finally, she underwent ORIF of her right mandibular body fracture using inferior border and tension band plates through an extraoral approach to control for lingual splay and ORIF of his left mandibular parasymphyseal fracture through an intraoral approach. Given the inherent benefit of the top–down approach and general avoidance of the condylar growth center, the displaced left subcondylar fracture was managed nonoperatively. Conventional titanium plate fixation systems were utilized. (*C*) Interval growth. CT imaging obtained at 12 years of age, nearly 6 years postoperatively demonstrates interval facial growth with significant healing and remodeling. Note removal of the lower midfacial fixation plates and mandibular tension bands at 8 years of age, approximately 2-year postoperatively. (*D*) Immediate postoperative dentition. Note the placement of inferior border plates along the mandible with monocortical fixation to avoid the developing dental follicles. Note the lack of consistent paranasal sinus aeration with unerupted maxillary dentition. Note the position of the displaced left subcondylar fracture, which was left to remodel. (*E*) Dental development into permanent dentition. At 12 years of age, nearly 6 years postoperatively, panoramic radiograph demonstrates extensive bony remodeling along the mandibular fractures with largely uninterrupted eruption of the permanent maxillary and mandibular dentition. Note some flattening of the left condylar head and mild vertical discrepancy along the ramus condyle unit.

deciduous period, case-by-case operative management during the mixed period, and closed versus open reduction and fixation during the permanent phase.[52]

In comparing the use of resorbable plate fixation to conventional titanium hardware, Chocron and colleagues found no differences in complication profiles.[54] It is our preference to utilize temporary traditional rigid fixation along the mandibular inferior border in a monocortical fashion to decrease injury to developing dentition (see Fig. 3D, E). Hardware is typically removed 8 to 12 weeks following fixation to prevent growth restriction and bony overgrowth.[5] Interdental control remains a challenge in the pediatric patient given a lack of fully erupted dentition, developing tooth buds, and/or loose, conical primary dentition that complicates conventional circumdental wiring techniques. Similar to maxillary wiring techniques, a lingual mandibular splint may be used to control splay using circumandibular wires.[5] If maxillomandibular fixation is needed, length of treatment should be less than 10 days followed by guiding elastics with functional therapy for an additional 10 days to decrease the risk of bony ankylosis.[5,55]

Bottom-Up/Inside–Out Approach

Unlike in the adult population where various operative approaches remain equally efficacious, the bottom–up/inside–out approach popularized by Markowitz and Manson may be more challenging.[4,37] The approach begins with the occlusal unit and frequently requires open reduction and internal fixation of displaced condylar fractures to restore lower posterior facial height and width, which is generally avoided in the pediatric population given the remodeling capacity of the condyle and its critical role as a growth center.[36] Moreover, the lack of erupted dentition may obviate the ability to obtain preoperative dental impressions and splints used to recreate the preinjury occlusion.

In the absence of mandibular condyle fractures and appropriate restoration of lower facial height, a bottom–up/inside–out approach may be considered.[4] Delena and colleagues reported the bottom–up approach as the second most common in their single institution retrospective review of pediatric panfacial fracture management.[4] Interdental control of the occlusal unit is critical in this approach because the remainder of the craniofacial skeleton builds on this foundation.[29] Mandibular splay from symphyseal and/or parasymphyseal fractures must be carefully reduced along the lingual cortex. Following reduction of the mandible and interdental control, the panfacial fracture articulates at the LeFort 1 level.[3,29,37] Next, the NOE segments are

overcorrected to correct the interorbital distance and to allow for the reduction of the ZMC fractures to restore appropriate facial width. The reduction of the NOE and ZMC segments is assessed along the temporal and (naso)frontal bones. Finally, the midfacial height is set by reducing the occlusal unit to the fixated upper midface with or without judicious autologous bone graft.

Soft Tissue Management and Postoperative Care

Despite limited subperiosteal dissection in the pediatric population, inadequate soft tissue redraping following degloving of the craniofacial skeleton results in soft tissue ptosis and the appearance of premature aging.[56] Resuspension of the soft tissues around the lower eyelid, malar eminence, and pterygomasseteric sling prevents the development of tear trough deformities and cicatricial scarring along orbital rim hardware, midface descent and nasolabial fold deepening, and jowling, respectively.[3,57] Temporal hollowing may be avoided by resuspension of the deep temporal fascia and meticulous dissection along the temporalis. Mentalis strain and chin ptosis can be avoided by resuspension of the mentalis. Canthal dystopia should be addressed with fixation of the lateral canthi in an overcorrected superior and posterior vector and fixation of the medial canthi in an overcorrected posterior and superior vector. Additionally, disruption of the medial canthus region warrants the use of external nasal bolster splints to compress and allow for readaptation of the medial canthus soft tissues and NOE fractures, respectively.[2]

Postoperative care largely follows adult fracture fixation protocols including a nonchew diet for 4 to 6 weeks, sinus precautions for 2 weeks, head of bed elevation greater than 30°, chlorhexidine oral rinses versus brushing in the setting of intraoral manipulation, and antibiotic ointment application along cutaneous incisions/lacerations. Vision checks and airway monitoring should be routinely performed.[3]

Complications

Beyond the site-specific complications that mirror the adult population, the most significant long-term consequence of pediatric fracture fixation remains its effect on subsequent growth and development. Rottgers and colleagues previously proposed a classification scheme of adverse outcomes following pediatric facial fracture repair.[58] Type 1 outcomes were defined as those related to the fracture itself, such as telecanthus following NOE fracture. Type 2 outcomes were defined as outcomes related to management, such as hardware infection. Type 3 outcomes were defined as outcomes related to impaired growth and development, such as midface hypoplasia. The authors further substantiated the prevailing pediatric fracture fixation theme in that nonoperative management is preferred to reduce the risk of Type 2 and 3 adverse outcomes.[4,5,9,39,58]

Growth disturbance following nasal trauma may occur due to premature ossification of the septovomerine suture.[9] Zygomatic fractures and fronto-orbital injuries after approximately 7 years of age (ie, radiographic evidence of frontal sinus pneumatization) traditionally do not lead to significant growth restriction.[9] NOE fractures may lead to compromised vertical and anterior-posterior growth of the midface.[9] Injury to the nasofrontal and frontomaxillary sutures and septum in displaced maxillary fractures is associated with midface hypoplasia requiring subsequent subcranial surgery.[59] Mandibular trauma, especially at the condyle, may result in malocclusion requiring orthognathic surgery at skeletal maturity.[39]

SUMMARY

Although rare, pediatric panfacial injuries typically result from high-energy mechanisms and lead to life-threatening polytrauma that requires an ATLS approach before facial fracture management. A systematic methodology to fracture reduction and fixation is essential to optimize immediate surgical outcomes and minimize future growth impairment. Although conservative management is preferred, there is equivocal evidence that primary surgical versus nonsurgical treatment leads to different rates of secondary surgery.

CLINICS CARE POINTS

- Panfacial trauma can be distracting injuries in critical ill patients. Follow standardized ATLS protocols during initial evaluation.
- Limit the extent of soft tissue and subperiosteal dissection needed to achieve the desired reduction/fixation, as wide undermining may lead to iatrogenic growth disturbance.
- Conventional titanium plating systems may be safely used to provide temporary rigid fixation for a period of 8 to 12 weeks without an increasing complication profile when compared with resorbable plating systems.
- Consider nonoperative management of nondisplaced or minimally displaced fractures given the extensive remodeling capacity of the pediatric patient. Consider operative management of displaced fractures to prevent the development of challenging end-stage deformities.
- Regardless of the management strategy used, counsel patients on the unpredictable need for secondary revision at skeletal maturity.

REFERENCES

1. Manson PN, Clark N, Robertson B, et al. Comprehensive management of pan-facial fractures. J Craniomaxillofac Trauma 1995;1(1):43–56.
2. Ali K, Lettieri SC. Management of Panfacial Fracture. Semin Plast Surg 2017;31(2):108–17.
3. Massenburg BB, Lang MS. Management of Panfacial Trauma: Sequencing and Pitfalls. Semin Plast Surg 2021;35(4):292–8.
4. Dalena MM, Liu FC, Halsey JN, et al. Assessment of Panfacial Fractures in the Pediatric Population. J Oral Maxillofac Surg 2020;78(7):1156–61.
5. Lim RB, Hopper RA. Pediatric Facial Fractures. Semin Plast Surg 2021;35(4):284–91.
6. Degala S, Sundar SS, Mamata KS. A Comparative Prospective Study of Two Different Treatment Sequences i.e. Bottom Up-Inside Out and Topdown-Outside in, in the Treatment of Panfacial Fractures. J Maxillofac Oral Surg 2015;14(4):986–94.
7. Suhaym O, Houle A, Griebel A, et al. The Quality of the Evidence in Craniomaxillofacial Trauma: Are We Making Progress? J Oral Maxillofac Surg 2021; 79(4):e891–7.
8. Imahara SD, Hopper RA, Wang J, et al. Patterns and outcomes of pediatric facial fractures in the United States: a survey of the National Trauma Data Bank. J Am Coll Surg 2008;207(5):710–6.
9. Singh DJ, Bartlett SP. Pediatric craniofacial fractures: long-term consequences. Clin Plast Surg 2004;31(3):499–518.
10. Moss ML, Salentijn L. The primary role of functional matrices in facial growth. Am J Orthod 1969;55(6):566–77.
11. Moss ML, Rankow RM. The role of the functional matrix in mandibular growth. Angle Orthod 1968;38(2):95–103.
12. Haug RH, Foss J. Maxillofacial injuries in the pediatric patient. Oral Surg Oral Med Oral Pathol Oral Radiol Endod 2000;90(2):126–34.
13. Fields HW. Craniofacial growth from infancy through adulthood. Background and clinical implications. Pediatr Clin North Am 1991;38(5):1053–88.
14. Enlow DH. Facial growth and development. Int J Oral Myol 1979;5(4):7–10.
15. Naran S, MacIsaac Z, Katzel E, et al. Pediatric Craniofacial Fractures: Trajectories and Ramifications. J Craniofac Surg 2016;27(6):1535–8.

16. Patterson R. The Le Fort fractures: Rene Le Fort and his work in anatomical pathology. Can J Surg 1991; 34(2):183–4.

17. Oji C. Fractures of the facial skeleton in children: a survey of patients under the age of 11 years. J Cranio-Maxillo-Fac Surg 1998;26(5):322–5.

18. Koltai PJ, Rabkin D. Management of facial trauma in children. Pediatr Clin North Am 1996;43(6):1253–75.

19. Kaban LB. Diagnosis and treatment of fractures of the facial bones in children 1943-1993. J Oral Maxillofac Surg 1993;51(7):722–9.

20. Totonchi A, Sweeney WM, Gosain AK. Distinguishing anatomic features of pediatric facial trauma. J Craniofac Surg 2012;23(3):793–8.

21. Braun TL, Xue AS, Maricevich RS. Differences in the Management of Pediatric Facial Trauma. Semin Plast Surg 2017;31(2):118–22.

22. Grunwaldt L, Smith DM, Zuckerbraun NS, et al. Pediatric facial fractures: demographics, injury patterns, and associated injuries in 772 consecutive patients. Plast Reconstr Surg 2011;128(6):1263–71.

23. McFadyen JG, Ramaiah R, Bhananker SM. Initial assessment and management of pediatric trauma patients. Int J Crit Illn Inj Sci 2012;2(3):121–7.

24. Andrew TW, Morbia R, Lorenz HP. Pediatric Facial Trauma. Clin Plast Surg 2019;46(2):239–47.

25. Ryan ML, Thorson CM, Otero CA, et al. Pediatric facial trauma: a review of guidelines for assessment, evaluation, and management in the emergency department. J Craniofac Surg 2011;22(4):1183–9.

26. Tung TC, Tseng WS, Chen CT, et al. Acute life-threatening injuries in facial fracture patients: a review of 1,025 patients. J Trauma 2000;49(3):420–4.

27. Mittal G, Mittal RK, Katyal S, et al. Airway management in maxillofacial trauma: do we really need tracheostomy/submental intubation. J Clin Diagn Res 2014;8(3):77–9.

28. Kita R, Kikuta T, Takahashi M, et al. Efficacy and complications of submental tracheal intubation compared with tracheostomy in maxillofacial trauma patients. J Oral Sci 2016;58(1):23–8.

29. Curtis W, Horswell BB. Panfacial fractures: an approach to management. Oral Maxillofac Surg Clin North Am 2013;25(4):649–60.

30. Zimmermann CE, Troulis MJ, Kaban LB. Pediatric facial fractures: recent advances in prevention, diagnosis and management. Int J Oral Maxillofac Surg 2006;35(1):2–13.

31. Alimohammadi R. Imaging of Dentoalveolar and Jaw Trauma. Radiol Clin North Am 2018;56(1):105–24.

32. Alcala-Galiano A, Arribas-Garcia IJ, Martin-Perez MA, et al. Pediatric facial fractures: children are not just small adults. Radiographics 2008; 28(2):441–61. quiz 618.

33. Gruss JS, Bubak PJ, Egbert MA. Craniofacial fractures. An algorithm to optimize results. Clin Plast Surg 1992;19(1):195–206.

34. Gruss JS, Phillips JH. Complex facial trauma: the evolving role of rigid fixation and immediate bone graft reconstruction. Clin Plast Surg 1989;16(1): 93–104.

35. He D, Zhang Y, Ellis E 3rd. Panfacial fractures: analysis of 33 cases treated late. J Oral Maxillofac Surg 2007;65(12):2459–65.

36. Yang R, Zhang C, Liu Y, et al. Why should we start from mandibular fractures in the treatment of panfacial fractures? J Oral Maxillofac Surg 2012;70(6): 1386–92.

37. Markowitz BL, Manson PN. Panfacial fractures: organization of treatment. Clin Plast Surg 1989;16(1): 105–14.

38. Vercler CJ, Sugg KB, Buchman SR. Split cranial bone grafting in children younger than 3 years old: debunking a surgical myth. Plast Reconstr Surg 2014;133(6):822e–7e.

39. Wheeler J, Phillips J. Pediatric facial fractures and potential long-term growth disturbances. Craniomaxillofac Trauma Reconstr 2011;4(1):43–52.

40. Yaremchuk MJ, Posnick JC. Resolving controversies related to plate and screw fixation in the growing craniofacial skeleton. J Craniofac Surg 1995;6(6): 525–38.

41. Rodriguez ED, Stanwix MG, Nam AJ, et al. Twenty-six-year experience treating frontal sinus fractures: a novel algorithm based on anatomical fracture pattern and failure of conventional techniques. Plast Reconstr Surg 2008;122(6):1850–66.

42. Coon D, Yuan N, Jones D, et al. Defining pediatric orbital roof fractures: patterns, sequelae, and indications for operation. Plast Reconstr Surg 2014;134(3): 442e–8e.

43. Firriolo JM, Ontiveros NC, Pike CM, et al. Pediatric Orbital Floor Fractures: Clinical and Radiological Predictors of Tissue Entrapment and the Effect of Operative Timing on Ocular Outcomes. J Craniofac Surg 2017;28(8):1966–71.

44. Broyles JM, Jones D, Bellamy J, et al. Pediatric Orbital Floor Fractures: Outcome Analysis of 72 Children with Orbital Floor Fractures. Plast Reconstr Surg 2015;136(4):822–8.

45. Grant JH 3rd, Patrinely JR, Weiss AH, et al. Trapdoor fracture of the orbit in a pediatric population. Plast Reconstr Surg 2002;109(2):482–9. discussion 490-485.

46. Azzi J, Azzi AJ, Cugno S. Resorbable Material for Pediatric Orbital Floor Reconstruction. J Craniofac Surg 2018;29(7):1693–6.

47. Markowitz BL, Manson PN, Sargent L, et al. Management of the medial canthal tendon in nasoethmoid orbital fractures: the importance of the central fragment in classification and treatment. Plast Reconstr Surg 1991;87(5):843–53.

48. Lopez J, Luck JD, Faateh M, et al. Pediatric Nasoorbitoethmoid Fractures: Cause, Classification, and

Management. Plast Reconstr Surg 2019;143(1): 211–22.

49. Chaudhry O, Isakson M, Franklin A, et al. Facial Fractures: Pearls and Perspectives. Plast Reconstr Surg 2018;141(5):742e–58e.

50. Davidson EH, Schuster L, Rottgers SA, et al. Severe Pediatric Midface Trauma: A Prospective Study of Growth and Development. J Craniofac Surg 2015; 26(5):1523–8.

51. Liao YF, Cole TJ, Mars M. Hard palate repair timing and facial growth in unilateral cleft lip and palate: a longitudinal study. Cleft Palate Craniofac J 2006;43(5):547–56.

52. Lopez J, Lake IV, Khavanin N, et al. Noninvasive Management of Pediatric Isolated, Condylar Fractures: Less Is More? Plast Reconstr Surg 2021; 147(2):443–52.

53. Smith DM, Bykowski MR, Cray JJ, et al. 215 mandible fractures in 120 children: demographics, treatment, outcomes, and early growth data. Plast Reconstr Surg 2013;131(6):1348–58.

54. Chocron Y, Azzi AJ, Davison P. Management of Pediatric Mandibular Fractures Using Resorbable Plates. J Craniofac Surg 2019;30(7):2111–4.

55. Bae SS, Aronovich S. Trauma to the Pediatric Temporomandibular Joint. Oral Maxillofac Surg Clin North Am 2018;30(1):47–60.

56. Phillips JH, Gruss JS, Wells MD, et al. Periosteal suspension of the lower eyelid and cheek following subciliary exposure of facial fractures. Plast Reconstr Surg 1991;88(1):145–8.

57. Hashem AM, Couto RA, Duraes EFR, et al. Facelift Part I: History, Anatomy, and Clinical Assessment. Aesthet Surg J 2020;40(1):1–18.

58. Rottgers SA, Decesare G, Chao M, et al. Outcomes in pediatric facial fractures: early follow-up in 177 children and classification scheme. J Craniofac Surg 2011;22(4):1260–5.

59. Ousterhout DK, Vargervik K. Maxillary hypoplasia secondary to midfacial trauma in childhood. Plast Reconstr Surg 1987;80(4):491–9.

Management of Soft Tissue Injuries in Children–A Comprehensive Review

Marcus Hwang, DDS, MD, Mark Engelstad, DDS, MD,
Srinivasa Rama Chandra, BDS, MD, FDS, FIBCSOMS*

KEYWORDS

- Pediatric trauma • Soft tissue injuries • Avulsion • Animal bite • Sports injuries • Facial injuries

KEY POINTS

- Pediatric soft tissue injuries may be severe but often present without an underlying fracture because of the significant pliability of the growing facial skeleton.
- Pediatric facial nerve and salivary duct injuries are similarly common like adult penetrating soft tissue injuries.
- Ocular and lacrimal system injuries are to be suspected in children and injury severity is higher compared with adults.
- Animal bites in children have a propensity to cause injury in the periocular subsite, another common cause being motor vehicle accidents.
- Airway examination and evaluation in children especially in penetrating injuries should be similar to adults; literature is sparse but injury sequela are commonly seen.

INTRODUCTION

Soft tissue injuries to the head and neck area in children is particularly challenging to manage, because these injuries can significantly affect the child's overall health and development. The management of such injuries requires a multidisciplinary approach involving surgical and nonsurgical interventions and close collaboration between health care professionals, parents, and caregivers. In this article, we review the various causes of injuries, specific considerations for each region of the head and neck, and approaches to the surgical management of soft tissue injuries in pediatric patients, including pharmacologic and nonpharmacologic therapies.

This article focuses on soft tissue injuries, and reviews specific anatomic regions. These include the scalp/forehead, periorbital region (eg, eyebrows, globe, canaliculi, lacrimal system), nose, cheeks, lips, ears, and neck/airway.

General Principles of Wound Management

The mechanisms of injuries in the pediatric population mimic those of adults and include motor vehicle accidents, trauma, assault, accidental injuries, falls, and others. Although most facial injuries in the pediatric population present without an underlying fracture, soft tissue injuries may be more severe in the pediatric population. Incomplete ossification of children protects the pediatric facial bones from fracture,[1,2] suggesting that blunt trauma may produce more devastating soft tissue injuries but without an underlying fracture. With increasing age, however, the risk for fracture increases by 14% with each additional year.[1,2] Nevertheless, clinical judgment and cause of injury should dictate the need for further imaging.

Facial injuries involve critical functional and esthetic considerations. Careful inspection should

Department of Oral Maxillofacial Surgery, Oregon Health and Sciences, Portland, OR, USA
* Corresponding author.
E-mail address: Ramachandra.srini@gmail.com

Oral Maxillofacial Surg Clin N Am 35 (2023) 619–629
https://doi.org/10.1016/j.coms.2023.06.003
1042-3699/23/

assess the involvement of the dermis, subcutaneous fat, musculature, nerves, and ducts. Findings should be documented. All wounds should be generously irrigated to prevent local infection and poor wound healing. Generally, layered closure with attention to the alignment of skin edges, hairlines, creases (nasolabial folds), and so forth should be considered. Underlying structures involving nerves, lacrimal system, and so forth should be adequately reviewed before repair. *Advanced Trauma Life Support* principles on trauma management are followed in extensive facial injuries, because airway, brain, and cervical spine injuries are correlated with trauma patterns. Isolated and single subsite facial injuries may not mandate a comprehensive trauma survey.

For the pediatric patient, compliance with repairing injuries in the emergency department may be complex and require treatment in the operating room. For wounds less than 4 cm in length and 0.5 cm in width, tissue adhesives (eg, Dermabond) may be an equivocal alternative to repairing superficial linear lacerations.[3] Additionally, tissue adhesives in these wounds can result in similar cosmetic outcomes when compared with wounds closed by sutures.[3] This is favorable in fearful patients with minor wounds that do not necessarily require general anesthesia for management.

Antibiotic Therapy

Soft tissue injuries of the face are common in children, with most being minor and requiring no more than simple wound care. Small superficial wounds do not require systemic oral antibiotics. But systemic oral antibiotics should be used in high-risk wounds, such as those contaminated with dirt or other foreign bodies, or in children with compromised immune systems.[4] Additionally, tetanus prophylaxis should be administered for contaminated wounds according to local protocols. Even for clean wounds, however, tetanus toxoid should be administered if the patient has had three or fewer doses or it has been more than 10 years since the last immunization (**Figs. 1** and **2**).[5]

SCALP/FOREHEAD
Background and Anatomic Considerations

Head injuries are devastating and cause significant mortality. Pediatric head injuries can have a high case fatality rate of 3.74.[6] Injuries to the scalp may result in traumatic brain injury and excessive blood loss, leading to subsequent hypovolemic shock. Injuries range from superficial abrasions to avulsions, often accompanied by skull fractures.

Pediatric skulls have open suture lines until undergoing ossification beginning approximately at

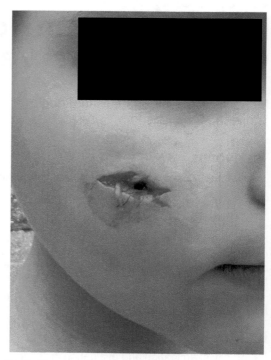

Fig. 1. Human bite injury of left cheek.

2 years of age. This is crucial because bones are freely mobile and may offer less brain protection against impact forces. Even puncture wounds from dog bites can often penetrate the soft tissue mantle and the underlying bones leading to an open injury.[7]

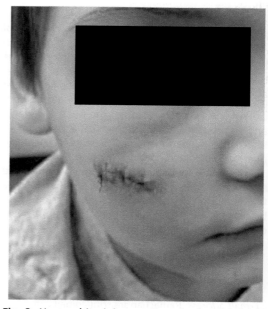

Fig. 2. Human bite injury postrepair complicated by localized infection.

The cause of most head injuries mimics those of the adult population and is secondary to motor vehicle accidents and falls. The prevalence of isolated scalp injuries without underlying fractures is unclear, because isolated studies are few (**Fig. 3**).[8]

The scalp is thick in infants and young children. This protects against injuries but is more susceptible to increased bleeding and swelling. The scalp comprises five layers, including the skin, subcutaneous tissue, galea aponeurotica (a dense fibrous layer), loose connective tissue, and the periosteum of the skull.

Rich arterial supply is from the external carotid artery branches, namely the superficial temporal, occipital, and posterior auricular arteries. However, its robust vascularity can lead to significant blood loss and hypovolemic shock if not controlled. The main vessels run along the galea aponeurotica, contributing to extensive blood loss because it is often disrupted.

The scalp is highly innervated and is supplied by branches of the trigeminal and cervical nerves. These sensory nerves travel through the subcutaneous tissue, which, when disrupted, can cause significant pain.

Hair typically obscures lacerations, making it difficult to assess the injury's extent accurately. It also acts as a nidus for dirt and debris, increasing the risk of infection.

Management

As with any injury event, a focused examination and comprehensive history should be taken. Moreover, depending on the clinical presentation and cause of the injury, noncontrast computed tomography (CT) should be obtained to assess underlying fractures and intracranial injury.[9] It may be difficult to thoroughly assess scalp wounds because of excessive hemorrhage, patient management, and the presence of hair and foreign bodies. Therefore, a thorough examination is

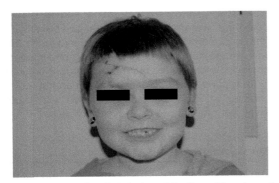

Fig. 3. Repair of scalp injuries with aligned borders of eyebrows.

best performed under general anesthesia before definitive management.[10]

Because of the scalp's highly vascular structure, uncontrolled hemorrhage can lead to hypovolemia and shock with more significant insults. Control of hemorrhage is crucial to prevent decompensation; arterial bleeds should be ligated timely, and compression should be applied through pressure dressings, and head wraps for hemostasis.

Simple lacerations may be repaired primarily in the emergency department under local anesthesia. However, most scalp wounds are difficult to examine because of the overlying hair and pain, so exploration may best be performed under general anesthesia. When exploring wounds and controlling bleeds, however, electrocautery should be used conservatively in the scalp to minimize damage to hair follicles and resultant alopecia.[9] Complex and avulsive lacerations require repair under general anesthesia and may require local flaps or skin grafts. Tissue expanders may be used for significant avulsive injuries. However, animal models have shown that pressure can cause deformation and erosion in growing facial bones, so we recommend avoiding its use in children younger than 3.[11]

AURICULAR
Background and Anatomic Considerations

Isolated ear injuries in the pediatric population are not well documented in the literature, although it accounts for 7% to 10% of emergency department visits yearly.[12] Injuries range from localized cellulitis, lacerations, and partial to avulsive injuries. A dread complication of auricular trauma is a postinjury or postoperative hematoma, leading to subsequent ear deformity, commonly called "cauliflower ear."

The ear canal is of external and internal contents. The external ear consists of elastic cartilage and acts as a hearing apparatus to direct acoustics through the middle ear for sound transmission by the inner ear. Blood supply to the ear is mainly from the superficial temporal artery and the posterior auricular artery, both arising from the external carotid artery. The neural sensation is from branches of the CN V, VII, and X and branches of spinal nerves C2 and C3.

Management

Auricles have excellent vascularity, and trauma can result in residual injuries with noticeable effects, even when it is hanging on a very thin pedicle if appropriately closed. Another consideration is that vascular tissue must cover all cartilage to avoid necrosis, which may be difficult in complex lacerations where devitalized tissue is removed. Local flaps or skin grafting from the contralateral ear may be helpful in such situations. After inspection of cartilage involvement, a three-layer closure is performed of the posterior skin, cartilage, and anterior skin. Cartilage is closed with clear 4–0 PDS, posterior skin is closed with absorbable sutures, and anterior/visible skin is closed with 5–0 Prolene or nylon sutures and removed in 5 to 7 days along with the overlying bolster dressing.[12]

PERIORBITAL REGION (EYEBROWS, EYELIDS, CANALICULI, LACRIMAL SYSTEM)
Background

The periorbital region compromises vital substructures that demand careful consideration. This section is subdivided to address the eyebrows, eyelids/conjunctiva, orbital contents (globe, extraocular muscles, periorbital fat, neurovascular bundles), and canaliculi/lacrimal system. For this review, the nose is not considered part of the periorbital region and is discussed later in this review.

When fractures are present in the periorbital region, they are often accompanied by more severe soft tissue injuries when compared with those of adults.[13] A study showed that 30% of patients with orbital fractures had concurrent periorbital and globe injuries.[14] They were also more likely to suffer orbital roof fractures because of immature form of the frontal sinus.[14,15]

Additionally, the injury pattern in this region differs between pediatric and adult populations. According to Hurst and colleagues,[16] children were two times more likely to suffer a periorbital injury from dog attacks when compared with adults. Stature, safety habits, and often reckless play are attributable to the differences in injury patterns and mechanisms among the young. Moreover, compared with other regions of the face, injuries to the periorbital region were more likely to require surgical correction in the operating room.[16] Nevertheless, the cause of periorbital injuries is diverse and includes animal bites, falls, assault, Gun shot wounds, and sports, the most common being motor vehicle accidents.[14]

Orbital Contents Considerations and Management (Globe, Extraocular Muscles, Lacrimal Gland, Periorbital Fat)

Injuries can range from minor corneal abrasions to globe rupture, the most common cause of blindness from orbital trauma. Fractures are associated with ophthalmologic emergencies, such as retinal detachment, vitreous hemorrhage, and optic nerve compression. Open globe injuries are one of the most devastating but are fortunately rare. Generally, globe injury following orbital trauma

ranges from 7.2% to 30%.[16] Given the significant morbidity, however, any suspicion of globe injury should warrant immediate ophthalmology consultation because it can lead to permanent vision loss.

It is well established that the most common reason for emergent surgical intervention in the orbital region is inferior rectus muscle entrapment secondary to orbital floor fracture.[14] Traumatic optic neuropathy can occur from any significant trauma to the orbits and is generally irreversible. Unfortunately, there is no substantial evidence that surgical intervention results in more favorable outcomes when compared with observation.[17–19]

Eyebrows Considerations and Management

If poorly managed, lacerations and avulsions of the eyebrows can have devastating esthetic results. The goal of repairing the eyebrows is to align the brows to the contralateral brow symmetrically. Although contamination and avulsions may obscure the eyebrows, it is recommended to avoid shaving if possible. The brows should be closed in layers, with the deeper orbicularis oculi addressed first. Superficially, the superior border should be aligned first, because alignment issues are more noticeable than those of the lower border.[20] If there are multiple injuries, it is advised to close the surrounding lacerations before closing the eyebrows to avoid tension that may distort the final esthetics.

Eyelids Considerations and Management

Special attention is needed in the management of eyelid injuries (Fig. 4). Poor wound management may lead to ptosis, lid retraction, scleral show, or persistent deformity that may persist or worsen through adolescent growth.[20] A retrospective review of eyelid lacerations in adults and children indicates that most complications are unrelated to the timing of repair, because many lacerations were repaired after 24 hours. Instead, complications, such as ptosis, lid retraction, and persistent deformity, were related to initial injury severity.[21] The most common cause of eyelid injuries is not well established. In patients with dog bite injuries, however, eyelids were the most commonly injured in the periorbital region.[16] As a general note, conjunctival injuries should be closed with knots away from the cornea to prevent irritation.[20]

Lacrimal/Canalicular Considerations and Management

The lacrimal duct apparatus is complex and merits a high degree of suspicion of injury whenever trauma involves the medial canthal region. Dog

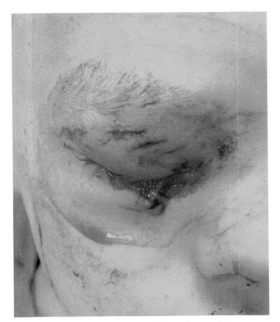

Fig. 4. Laceration injury involving the eyelids.

bites are the most common cause for lacrimal injuries, but fortunately, lacrimal sac and nasolacrimal duct involvement is rare.[22] Murchison and Bilyk[23] reviewed 137 lacrimal system injuries and found that most were isolated lacrimal insults. Diagnosis is made by inspection and careful probing under general anesthesia. If the injury is suspected, the severed ends should be identified and realigned. They are repaired by using a silastic catheter or Crawford tube to align the proximal and distal ends. Severe complications include persistent epiphora, esthetic deformity, and dacrocystitis.

NASAL REGION
Background and Anatomic Considerations

Injuries to the nose range from simple lacerations to total avulsions and requires special consideration in the pediatric population. One such consideration is the two growth areas of cartilage-bony interfaces (eg, septal cartilage) to prevent halting or disruption of midface growth.[24,25] If injured, this could result in decreased projection or asymmetries during the two postnatal growth spurts: early childhood and puberty.

When compared with those of adults, the pediatric nose is supported by cartilage because the nasal bones have incomplete ossification and open sutures lines. The soft, compliant cartilage bends easily during blunt trauma, and the pliable nasal bones are more prone to greenstick fractures when compared with adults.[25] Given this

pliability of the nasal structure, even in the absence of a fracture, there is an increased risk for soft tissue disruption and subsequent hematoma.[26] Therefore, septal hematomas were observed to be more common in the pediatric population compared with adults.[26] Septal hematoma is an untreated surgical emergency that can result in avascular necrosis.

Management

The overall goal in repair is to reestablish the premorbid shape and function while preventing subsequent revisions. It is common, however, for nose injuries in pediatric populations to require revisions because of the disruption of growth plates. Immerman and colleagues[27] recommended allowing complete healing before revision, and it was shown that the healing period could range from 6 to 24 months.

Nasal soft tissue injuries should be cleansed, irrigated, and primarily repaired. Full-thickness injuries should be repaired in a layered technique, starting deep and working superficial. Cartilage should be repaired first and done with permanent or slow-absorbing sutures. This reestablishes the proper framework to support the overlying soft tissue. Deep tissue should be repaired with sutures with prolonged absorption, and the nasal mucosa should be repaired with a fine, fast-absorbing suture. Finally, any skin defects should be closed with a fine, nonresorbable or absorbable suture or tissue adhesive, depending on the patient's age.

CHEEK
Background and Anatomic Considerations

The cheek is defined as the region below the eyes and between the nose and ears. This region comprises a large percentage of the face, because it is also bilateral. This region consists of eight muscles shown in **Fig. 5**. Lacerations and avulsive injuries are often caused by sharp, penetrating trauma.[28] It was shown by Hurst and colleagues[16] that this region was the most commonly injured subunit of the central target area (ie, lips, nose, cheeks) from traumatic dog bites.

The cheek comprises most of the facial fat pads and provides the most volume. Injury to these areas can cause significant asymmetry and lack of facial fullness.[29] Branches of the facial and trigeminal nerves innervate the skin and muscles of the cheek. After exiting the stylohyoid foramen, the facial nerve arises from the parotid gland to branch into five main branches to provide motor innervation to the facial muscles. The trigeminal nerve divides into three main branches, providing

Muscles located in the cheek region:

- Orbicularis oculi muscle (lower border)

- Levator labii superioris muscle

- Levator labii superioris alaeque nasi muscle

- Risorius muscle

- Levator anguli oris muscle

- Zygomaticus major and minor muscles

- Buccinator muscle

- Masseter muscle

Fig. 5. Muscles of the cheek.

sensation to the entire face and motor function to the masseter (**Figs. 6–12**).

Numerous muscles in this region are responsible for facial expression, mastication, and speaking. Lastly, the facial artery and subsequent branches provide a significant blood supply to this region.

The parotid duct facilitates the flow of saliva from the parotid salivary glands to the oral cavity. It originates at the gland, and travels superficially to the master before piercing through the buccinator and terminating intraorally. Clinicians should

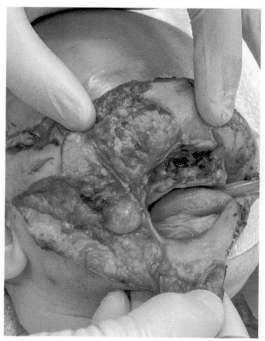

Fig. 7. Extraoral and intraoral lacerations in continuity.

accurately assess and document parotid duct injuries, which are often not diagnosed during the initial evaluation.[30,31]

Management

Facial expression, asymmetry, and nerve sensation should be accurately documented before wound exploration and repair. Subsequently, management depends on the structures previously mentioned. Injuries can range from minor abrasions, convulsions, varying thickness of lacerations with often communication to the oral cavity, avulsive injuries, trigeminal (V1) and facial nerve injuries, and parotid salivary duct injuries.

As with other injuries, adequate removal of foreign bodies, debridement, and irrigation should be performed. Vascular injuries should be microsurgically repaired, and soft tissue injuries should be closed in layers with resorbable sutures. Care should be undertaken to avoid unnecessary removal of the facial fat pads to avoid poor cosmesis.

If injury to the parotid duct is suspected, the orifice of Stensen may be probed in the operating room under general anesthesia.[32] If an injury is missed and proper repair is not achieved, it may lead to debilitating facial fistulas or sialoceles.[32] Cannulation is safely performed with a lacrimal probe or an angiocatheter (20–22 gauge)

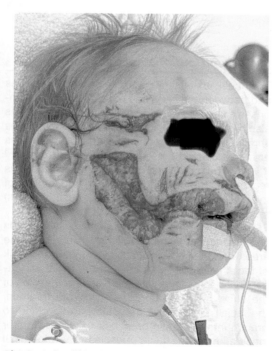

Fig. 6. Animal bite injury to oral structures and cheek.

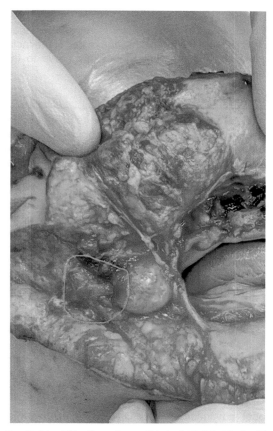

Fig. 8. Identification of parotid duct highlighted with the *green circular* marker

intraorally through the distal end of the Stensen orifice to assess for tract compromise. If saline can be transmitted through the catheter to the outer side, this would confirm an injury to the duct. The anastomosis is performed to reapproximate the severed portions of the duct, with the placement of an intraluminal stent to prevent stenosis, and it is removed after 10 to 14 days (**Fig. 13**).

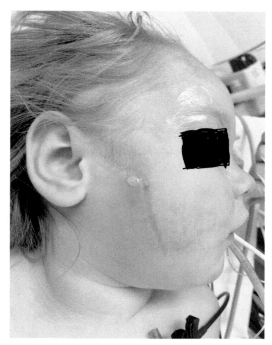

Fig. 10. Scars healing well, complicated by cutaneous salivary fistula with continued salivary drainage.

Other options include autologous venous grafts.[33] In situations where the distal end cannot be located or is avulsed, diverting the proximal end to a new location intraorally may be necessary and sutured with 8–0 nylon. In severe injuries that require ligation of the remaining duct, symptomatic management should be pursued during the period in which the parotid gland atrophies. This is accomplished with warm compresses and anti-sialagogue medications. Postoperatively, sialography should be considered even with successful repair to assess long-term outcomes.

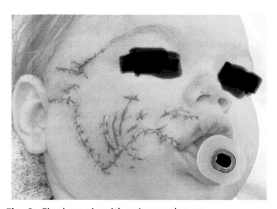

Fig. 9. Final repair with primary closure.

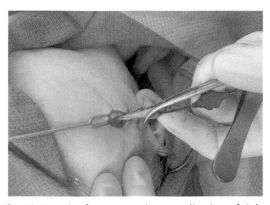

Fig. 11. Repair of postoperative complication of sialocele and cutaneous fistula.

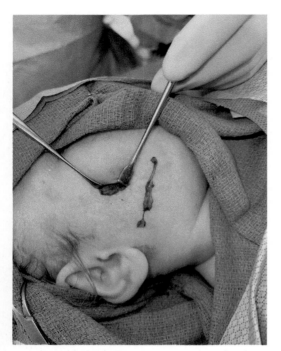

Fig. 12. Fistulectomy and removal of ductal tract.

LIPS
Background and Anatomic Considerations

Lip and intraoral injuries are common in the pediatric population and can result from various trauma etiologies. Avulsive injuries are most common from animal bite injuries. The lips are divided into the upper and lower lips, with the underlying orbicularis oris muscle as the significant musculature. Blood supply is from the branches of the facial

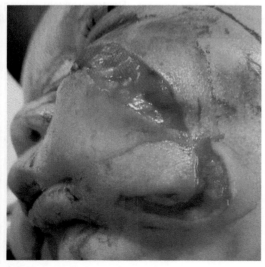

Fig. 13. Deep laceration with concern for facial nerve and parotid duct injury.

artery, and neural sensation is from V2 and V3 to the upper and lower lips, respectively. Motor innervation is from the buccal branch motor of the facial nerve and the marginal mandibular nerve to the upper and lower lips, respectively.

Management

Injuries to the lip require attention to proper alignment to prevent easily identifiable defects after repair, the most critical landmarks being the vermilion border, Cupid's bow, and philtral columns.[12]

Generally, injuries should be repaired from inside out and primary closure is achievable as long as only less than one-third of the lip is missing. Oral injuries (teeth, gingiva, mucosa) should be repaired as necessary first. Injuries involving the inner mucosa layer should be closed. A key stitch is then placed to reapproximate the vermilion to ensure proper alignment. Absorbable 4–0 braided sutures should reapproximate the underlying orbicularis, the mucosa is closed with 4–0 chromic gut sutures, and the skin is closed with 5–0 fast-absorbing monofilament or permanent sutures. Proper closure in layers is essential to provide proper function and prevent muscle bulging after recovery.[34]

Most lacerations are closed primarily or with local advancement flaps. Avulsive injuries that involved more than one-third of the lip may require more complex reconstruction, such as local, rotational flaps or free flaps, but is beyond the scope of this review and is rare in the pediatric population.

NECK/AIRWAY
Background and Anatomic Considerations

A penetrating neck injury is defined as one that breaches the platysma muscle, because underlying this layer are the major neck vessels. Multiple retrospective studies found that such injuries are uncommon in the pediatric population.[35–39] However, despite the rarity, the mortality rate is high (6%–40%) and suggests that such injuries can be devastating.[35,38,39] Other complications include airway emergencies, vascular and neurologic compromise, and aerodigestive injuries, all of which can worsen the acute and long-term postinsult course. To our knowledge, there is no comprehensive review of the literature regarding neck injuries in the pediatric population and, thus, no established algorithm for intervention workflow in penetrating neck injuries (**Fig. 14**).

The neck is classically divided into three zones. Zone I is bordered between the clavicles/sternum to the cricoid cartilage. Zone II is bordered by the cricoid cartilage to the angle of the mandible.

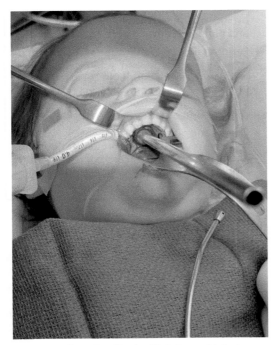

Fig. 14. Intubated patient with intraoral injuries.

Zone III spans from superior to the angle of the mandible to the skull base. Most injuries to the neck in the adult and pediatric population occur in zone II.[35,38,39] The mechanism of injuries varies in the literature but the most common are those secondary to Motor Vehicle Collisions or penetrating injuries.[35,38,40] Animal bites are disastrous but less common than those of assault. Unsurprisingly, projectile/missile wounds typically from foul play and assault occurs more often in older children, whereas animal bites are more common in younger children.[38,40]

Management

It is important to decide whether observation versus surgical exploration is warranted in the injured pediatric patient. The options for management include examination, laryngoscopy, barium swallow, CT with contrast, or CT angiogram. These diagnostic work-ups aid in determining the need for an invasive and traumatic surgical exploration, which have been shown to increase hospital length stay.[39,40] There is no general consensus, however, on which physical examination findings should prompt a mandatory versus selective exploration. Despite using penetration of the platysma as an indication for surgical exploration, most attempts resulted in negative findings.[40] In one study, 18 of 39 (46%) with platysma injury underwent exploration, but 15 of 18 (83.3%) had negative findings.[10,40]

The work-up for penetrating neck injuries remains erratic and varies depending on the

Table 1
Facial scar management in children and safety profile

Surgical Scar Interventions	Medical Therapy	Laser and Multimodal Therapy
Scar revision: Z- or W-plasty; morbidity of additional surgery	5-Fluorouracil efficacy and safety not established in children	CO_2 laser 500 nm
Scar excision: keloids and hypertrophic scars to increase range of facial animation; recurrence rate is high and additional procedures	Corticosteroids: direct injections in hypertrophic and keloid scars; triamcinolone acetonide 40 mg/mL; scar atrophy, recurrence, benzyl alcohol carrier-related toxicity for neonates	Pulsed dye laser 595 nm: hypervascular lesions
Fat transfers and grafting: atrophic scars; growth changes and additional procedures adds to children's distress	Matrix metalloproteinase-1	Laser-assisted drug delivery by fractional photothermolysis elimination and increased absorption
Dermabrasion: not advised in children, adolescents may tolerate well	Fibroblastic activity inhibitors, such as dipeptidyl-peptidase IV	Pigment elimination by Nd-YAG lasers
	Stem cell; interleukin-10; fibroblast growth factor	

Adapted from Krakowski AC, Totri CR, Donelan MB, Shumaker PR. Scar Management in the Pediatric and Adolescent Populations. Pediatrics. 2016;137(2):e20142065.

specialist or attending-on-call.[35] Generally, wound exploration is performed in deep lacerations, those near the major neck vessels, or those who exhibit hemodynamic instability.[35–39] Many authors advocate that the major indications for mandatory exploration should include (1) continued bleeding from a wound, hematoma, shock; (2) blood in the aerodigestive tract; (3) subcutaneous emphysema; (4) neurologic deficits; and (5) inability to accurately access the patient.[36,37,39] Unfortunately, no established guidelines exist for surgical exploration, which remains controversial among trauma surgeons (**Table 1**).

Pediatric patients generally heal well and thus scar revision is reserved if conservative measures fail or if the scar affects function and appearance. Revisions are typically needed if they involve delicate regions with thin tissues, such as the eyelids, and esthetics borders.[41,42]

Conservative therapy aims to reduce the appearance of scars, improve function, and prevent or minimize the risk of hypertrophic or keloid scarring. 5-Fluorouracil and Kenalog injections are typically used in the adult population for scar management, but generally not recommended for pediatric patients. Laser therapies tend to have better results in children when compared with adults because pigmented and vascular lesions become more resistant with age.[41] Generally, the pulsed dye laser is the preferred option. Other well-tolerated options include vitamin E–based petroleum, silicone-based patches, or dermabrasion. Dermabrasion has been studied in pediatric burn patients but has not been extensively studied in trauma patients.

CLINICS CARE POINTS

- During external ear repair in children, the base and projection of the ear should be in three dimensional symmetry to the contralateral side, and should not be advanced or rotated.
- Fluid management and volume resuscitation is critical in burns, soft tissue injury associated bleeds in scalp and perioral subsites of pediatric patients as volume associated shock can be acute.
- Review, repair and dressing in children may need some mild to moderate sedation for anxiolysis and compliance.
- Children had more severe soft tissue injuries Compared to adults with similar periorbital fractures, as Only 30% of children with

orbital fractures had concurrent periorbital and globe injuries.
- Periorbital injury pattern facial region differs between pediatric and adult populations. With more severe injuries in children. As children were two times more likely to suffer a periorbital injury from dog attacks when compared to adults.
- Orbital and globe injury incidence is 7- 30% in children, lower than adults but inferior rectus entrapment is more common than direct globe penetrative injury due to green stick fracture of orbital floor.

REFERENCES

1. Gassner R, Tuli T, Hächl O, et al. Craniomaxillofacial trauma in children: a review of 3,385 cases with 6,060 injuries in 10 years. J Oral Maxillofac Surg 2004;62(4):399–407.
2. Zhou HH, Lv K, Rong T, et al. Maxillofacial injuries in pediatric patients. J Craniofac Surg 2021;32(4): 1476–9.
3. Quinn JV, Drzewiecki A, Li MM, et al. A randomized, controlled trial comparing a tissue adhesive with suturing in the repair of pediatric facial lacerations. Ann Emerg Med 1993;22(7):1130–5.
4. Cummings P, Del Beccaro MA. Antibiotics to prevent infection of simple wounds: a meta-analysis of randomized studies. Am J Emerg Med 1995;13(4): 396–400.
5. Black KD, Cico SJ, Caglar D. Wound management. Pediatr Rev 2015;36(5):207–15 [quiz: 16].
6. National Trauma Data Bank 2016 Pediatric Annual Report 2016. Available at: https://www.facs.org/media/d3ufvsmy/ntdb-pediatric-annual-report-2016.pdf. Accessed July 23, 2023.
7. Mason AC, Zabel DD, Manders EK. Occult craniocerebral injuries from dog bites in young children. Ann Plast Surg 2000;45(5):531–4.
8. Da Dalt L, Marchi AG, Laudizi L, et al. Predictors of intracranial injuries in children after blunt head trauma. Eur J Pediatr 2006;165(3):142–8.
9. Horswell BB, Jaskolka MS. Pediatric head injuries. Oral Maxillofac Surg Clin North Am 2012;24(3): 337–50.
10. Chandra SR, Zemplenyi KS. Issues in pediatric craniofacial trauma. Facial Plast Surg Clin North Am 2017;25(4):581–91.
11. Schmelzeisen R, Schimming R, Schwipper V, et al. Influence of tissue expanders on the growing craniofacial skeleton. J Cranio-Maxillo-Fac Surg 1999; 27(3):153–9.
12. Zimmerman ZA, Sidle DM. Soft tissue injuries including auricular hematoma management. Facial Plast Surg Clin North Am 2022;30(1):15–22.

13. Luce EA. Discussion: pediatric orbital floor fractures: outcome analysis of 72 children with orbital floor fractures. Plast Reconstr Surg 2015;136(4):829–30.

14. Halsey J, Argüello-Angarita M, Carrasquillo OY, et al. Periorbital and globe injuries in pediatric orbital fractures: a retrospective review of 116 patients at a level 1 trauma center. Craniomaxillofac Trauma Reconstr 2021;14(3):183–8.

15. Cossman JP, Morrison CS, Taylor HO, et al. Traumatic orbital roof fractures: interdisciplinary evaluation and management. Plast Reconstr Surg 2014;133(3):335e–43e.

16. Hurst PJ, Hoon Hwang MJ, Dodson TB, et al. Children have an increased risk of periorbital dog bite injuries. J Oral Maxillofac Surg 2020;78(1):91–100.

17. Yu-Wai-Man P, Griffiths PG. Surgery for traumatic optic neuropathy. Cochrane Database Syst Rev 2013;6(6):Cd005024.

18. Goldenberg-Cohen N, Miller NR, Repka MX. Traumatic optic neuropathy in children and adolescents. J aapos 2004;8(1):20–7.

19. Kashkouli MB, Yousefi S, Nojomi M, et al. Traumatic Optic Neuropathy Treatment Trial (TONTT): open label, phase 3, multicenter, semi-experimental trial. Graefes Arch Clin Exp Ophthalmol 2018;256(1):209–18.

20. Vasconez HC, Buseman JL, Cunningham LL. Management of facial soft tissue injuries in children. J Craniofac Surg 2011;22(4):1320–6.

21. Chiang E, Bee C, Harris GJ, et al. Does delayed repair of eyelid lacerations compromise outcome? Am J Emerg Med 2017;35(11):1766–7.

22. Ducasse A, Arndt C, Brugniart C, et al. [Lacrimal traumatology]. J Fr Ophtalmol 2016;39(2):213–8.

23. Murchison AP, Bilyk JR. Pediatric canalicular lacerations: epidemiology and variables affecting repair success. J Pediatr Ophthalmol Strabismus 2014;51(4):242–8.

24. Basa K, Ezzat WH. Soft tissue trauma to the nose: management and special considerations. Facial Plast Surg 2021;37(4):473–9.

25. Wright RJ, Murakami CS, Ambro BT. Pediatric nasal injuries and management. Facial Plast Surg 2011;27(5):483–90.

26. Javaid M, Feldberg L, Gipson M. Primary repair of dog bites to the face: 40 cases. J R Soc Med 1998;91(8):414–6.

27. Immerman S, Constantinides M, Pribitkin EA, et al. Nasal soft tissue trauma and management. Facial Plast Surg 2010;26(6):522–31.

28. Hemenway WG, Bergstrom L. Parotid duct fistula: a review. South Med J 1971;64(8):912–8.

29. Nguyen JD DH. Anatomy, Head and Neck, Cheeks. Updated 2022 Aug 8. In: StatPearls Internet. Treasure Island (FL): StatPearls Publishing; 2022 Jan-. Available from: https://www.ncbi.nlm.nih.gov/books/NBK546659/.

30. Abramson M. Treatment of parotid duct injuries. Laryngoscope 1973;83(11):1764–8.

31. DeVylder J, Carlo J, Stratigos GT. Early recognition and treatment of the traumatically transected parotid duct: report of case. J Oral Surg 1978;36(1):43–4.

32. Steinberg MJ, Herréra AF. Management of parotid duct injuries. Oral Surg Oral Med Oral Pathol Oral Radiol Endod 2005;99(2):136–41.

33. Chudakov O, Ludchik T. Microsurgical repair of Stensen's & Wharton's ducts with autogenous venous grafts. An experimental study on dogs. Int J Oral Maxillofac Surg 1999;28(1):70–3.

34. Farrior RT, Jarchow RC, Rojas B. Primary and late plastic repair of soft tissue injuries. Otolaryngol Clin North Am 1983;16(3):697–708.

35. Abujamra L, Joseph MM. Penetrating neck injuries in children: a retrospective review. Pediatr Emerg Care 2003;19(5):308–13.

36. Hall JR, Reyes HM, Meller JL. Penetrating zone-II neck injuries in children. J Trauma 1991;31(12):1614–7.

37. Martin WS, Gussack GS. Pediatric penetrating head and neck trauma. Laryngoscope 1990;100(12):1288–91.

38. Mutabagani KH, Beaver BL, Cooney DR, et al. Penetrating neck trauma in children: a reappraisal. J Pediatr Surg 1995;30(2):341–4.

39. Kim MK, Buckman R, Szeremeta W. Penetrating neck trauma in children: an urban hospital's experience. Otolaryngol Head Neck Surg 2000;123(4):439–43.

40. Vick LR, Islam S. Adding insult to injury: neck exploration for penetrating pediatric neck trauma. Am Surg 2008;74(11):1104–6.

41. Mobley SR, Sjogren PP. Soft tissue trauma and scar revision. Facial Plast Surg Clin North Am 2014;22(4):639–51.

42. Krakowski AC, Totri CR, Donelan MB, et al. Scar management in the pediatric and adolescent populations. Pediatrics 2016;137(2):e20142065.

UNITED STATES POSTAL SERVICE®

Statement of Ownership, Management, and Circulation (All Periodicals Publications Except Requester Publications)

1. Publication Title ORAL & MAXILLOFACIAL SURGERY CLINICS OF NORTH AMERICA	**2. Publication Number** 006 – 362
	3. Filing Date 9/18/2023
4. Issue Frequency FEB, MAY, AUG, NOV	**5. Number of Issues Published Annually** 4
	6. Annual Subscription Price $409.00

7. Complete Mailing Address of Known Office of Publication *(Not printer)* *(Street, city, county, state, and ZIP+4®)*
ELSEVIER INC.
230 Park Avenue, Suite 800
New York, NY 10169

Contact Person
Malathi Samayan
Telephone *(Include area code)*
91-44-4299-4507

8. Complete Mailing Address of Headquarters or General Business Office of Publisher *(Not printer)*
ELSEVIER INC.
230 Park Avenue, Suite 800
New York, NY 10169

9. Full Names and Complete Mailing Addresses of Publisher, Editor, and Managing Editor *(Do not leave blank)*

Publisher *(Name and complete mailing address)*
Dolores Meloni, ELSEVIER INC.
1600 JOHN F KENNEDY BLVD. SUITE 1600
PHILADELPHIA, PA 19103-2899

Editor *(Name and complete mailing address)*
JOHN VASSALLO, ELSEVIER INC.
1600 JOHN F KENNEDY BLVD. SUITE 1600
PHILADELPHIA, PA 19103-2899

Managing Editor *(Name and complete mailing address)*
PATRICK MANLEY, ELSEVIER INC.
1600 JOHN F KENNEDY BLVD. SUITE 1600
PHILADELPHIA, PA 19103-2899

10. Owner *(Do not leave blank. If the publication is owned by a corporation, give the name and address of the corporation immediately followed by the names and addresses of all stockholders owning or holding 1 percent or more of the total amount of stock. If not owned by a corporation, give the names and addresses of the individual owners. If owned by a partnership or other unincorporated firm, give its name and address as well as those of each individual owner. If the publication is published by a nonprofit organization, give its name and address.)*

Full Name	Complete Mailing Address
WHOLLY OWNED SUBSIDIARY OF REED/ELSEVIER, US HOLDINGS	1600 JOHN F KENNEDY BLVD. SUITE 1600 PHILADELPHIA, PA 19103-2899

11. Known Bondholders, Mortgagees, and Other Security Holders Owning or Holding 1 Percent or More of Total Amount of Bonds, Mortgages, or Other Securities. If none, check box ► ☐ None

Full Name	Complete Mailing Address
N/A	

12. Tax Status *(For completion by nonprofit organizations authorized to mail at nonprofit rates)* *(Check one)*
The purpose, function, and nonprofit status of this organization and the exempt status for federal income tax purposes:
☒ Has Not Changed During Preceding 12 Months
☐ Has Changed During Preceding 12 Months *(Publisher must submit explanation of change with this statement)*

PS Form **3526**, July 2014 *(Page 1 of 4 (see instructions page 4))* PSN: 7530-01-000-9931   PRIVACY NOTICE: See our privacy policy on www.usps.com.

---

13. Publication Title ORAL & MAXILLOFACIAL SURGERY CLINICS OF NORTH AMERICA				**14. Issue Date for Circulation Data Below** AUGUST 2023

15. Extent and Nature of Circulation			**Average No. Copies Each Issue During Preceding 12 Months**	**No. Copies of Single Issue Published Nearest to Filing Date**
a. Total Number of Copies *(Net press run)*			402	386
b. Paid Circulation *(By Mail and Outside the Mail)*	(1)	Mailed Outside-County Paid Subscriptions Stated on PS Form 3541 *(Include paid distribution above nominal rate, advertiser's proof copies, and exchange copies)*	322	317
	(2)	Mailed In-County Paid Subscriptions Stated on PS Form 3541 *(Include paid distribution above nominal rate, advertiser's proof copies, and exchange copies)*	0	0
	(3)	Paid Distribution Outside the Mails Including Sales Through Dealers and Carriers, Street Vendors, Counter Sales, and Other Paid Distribution Outside USPS®	60	54
	(4)	Paid Distribution by Other Classes of Mail Through the USPS *(e.g., First-Class Mail®)*	13	8
c. Total Paid Distribution *(Sum of 15b (1), (2), (3), and (4))* ►			395	379
d. Free or Nominal Rate Distribution *(By Mail and Outside the Mail)*	(1)	Free or Nominal Rate Outside-County Copies Included on PS Form 3541	6	6
	(2)	Free or Nominal Rate In-County Copies Included on PS Form 3541	0	0
	(3)	Free or Nominal Rate Copies Mailed at Other Classes Through the USPS *(e.g., First-Class Mail)*	0	0
	(4)	Free or Nominal Rate Distribution Outside the Mail *(Carriers or other means)*	1	1
e. Total Free or Nominal Rate Distribution *(Sum of 15d (1), (2), (3) and (4))* ►			7	7
f. Total Distribution *(Sum of 15c and 15e)* ►			402	386
g. Copies not Distributed *(See Instructions to Publishers #4 (page #3))* ►			0	0
h. Total *(Sum of 15f and g)* ►			402	386
i. Percent Paid *(15c divided by 15f times 100)* ►			98.26%	98.19%

* If you are claiming electronic copies, go to line 16 on page 3. If you are not claiming electronic copies, skip to line 17 on page 3.

PS Form 3526, July 2014 (Page 2 of 4)

16. Electronic Copy Circulation	**Average No. Copies Each Issue During Preceding 12 Months**	**No. Copies of Single Issue Published Nearest to Filing Date**
a. Paid Electronic Copies ►		
b. Total Paid Print Copies (Line 15c) + Paid Electronic Copies (Line 16a) ►		
c. Total Print Distribution (Line 15f) + Paid Electronic Copies (Line 16a) ►		
d. Percent Paid (Both Print & Electronic Copies) (16b divided by 16c × 100) ►		

☒ **I certify that 50% of all my distributed copies (electronic and print) are paid above a nominal price.**

17. Publication of Statement of Ownership
☒ If the publication is a general publication, publication of this statement is required. Will be printed
in the NOVEMBER 2023 issue of this publication.   ☐ Publication not required.

18. Signature and Title of Editor, Publisher, Business Manager, or Owner

Malathi Samayan   Date 9/18/2023

Malathi Samayan - Distribution Controller

I certify that all information furnished on this form is true and complete. I understand that anyone who furnishes false or misleading information on this form or who omits material or information requested on the form may be subject to criminal sanctions (including fines and imprisonment) and/or civil sanctions (including civil penalties).

PS Form **3526**, July 2014 *(Page 3 of 4)*   PRIVACY NOTICE: See our privacy policy on www.usps.com.

Moving?

Make sure your subscription moves with you!

To notify us of your new address, find your **Clinics Account Number** (located on your mailing label above your name), and contact customer service at:

Email: journalscustomerservice-usa@elsevier.com

800-654-2452 (subscribers in the U.S. & Canada)
314-447-8871 (subscribers outside of the U.S. & Canada)

Fax number: 314-447-8029

Elsevier Health Sciences Division
Subscription Customer Service
3251 Riverport Lane
Maryland Heights, MO 63043

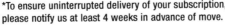

9780443182808